LECTURES ON THE

THYROID

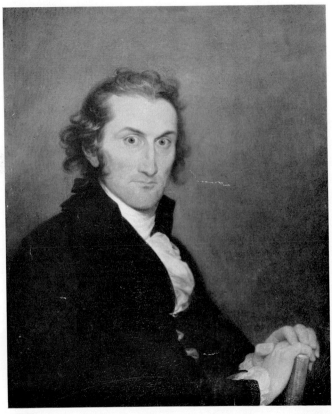

Portrait of Dr. Lemuel Hopkins (1750–1801), physician of Hartford, by John Trumbull. Dr. Hopkins's eyes show unmistakable evidence of his having, or having had, Graves's disease. (Courtesy of Yale University Art Gallery.)

LECTURES ON THE

THYROID

BY

J. H. MEANS, M.D.

Jackson Professor of Clinical Medicine Emeritus
Harvard University
Former Chief of Medical Services, Massachusetts General Hospital
Physician, Massachusetts Institute of Technology

HARVARD UNIVERSITY PRESS · CAMBRIDGE

1954

Distributed in Great Britain by
GEOFFREY CUMBERLEGE
Oxford University Press
London

Library of Congress Catalog Card Number 54–5021

Printed in the United States of America

TO ALL MY COLLEAGUES

OF THE THYROID CLINIC

OF THE

MASSACHUSETTS GENERAL HOSPITAL

PREFACE

The lectures collected in this volume were delivered in various places during the period from June 1949 to April 1953. Although not in any way planned as a sequential course, the several lectures yet have some relevancy one to another. The excuse for publishing them in the present form is that, taken together, they epitomize some of the thoughts which I have derived from my own work on the thyroid, together with that of many brilliant colleagues, whose brains I have freely picked. In my own case the experience has extended over some forty years. The collection is a personal account. It is not intended in any sense as a complete coverage of the topics discussed.

The first four lectures, previously published in medical journals, have all been carefully edited and brought up to present knowledge as nearly as possible by means of textual alterations. In the doing of this I have had the invaluable aid and advice of Dr. John B. Stanbury, my successor in the Thyroid Clinic at the Massachusetts General Hospital.

Lecture I was the third annual Harvard Lecture given at the University of Colorado Medical Center, Denver, on December 8, 1950, under the auspices of the Rocky Mountain Harvard Medical Alumni Association.

Lectures II and III were the seventeenth course of lectures under the William Sydney Thayer and Susan Read Thayer Lectureship in Clinical Medicine. They were delivered at the Johns Hopkins Hospital, Baltimore, on April 26 and 27, 1951.

Lecture IV was the Holme Lecture delivered at University College Hospital Medical School, London, on June 23, 1949.

Lecture V was the Hanau W. Loeb Lecture of the Alphi Pi

Chapter of Phi Delta Epsilon, St. Louis University School of Medicine, delivered on March 26, 1953.

I am grateful for permission to republish to the *Annals of Internal Medicine* in the case of Lecture I, the *Bulletin of the Johns Hopkins Hospital* in that of Lectures II and III, the *Lancet* for Lecture IV, and the *Medical Bulletin of St. Louis University* in the case of Lecture V.

J. H. MEANS

CONTENTS

LECTURES ON THE

THYROID

1 The integrative action of the endocrine system

For the subject of this lecture I have chosen certain aspects of the fundamental question, "What makes us tick?"

"What makes us tick as human beings" is perhaps relatively easy to answer. We might say the cerebral cortex or, if you prefer, the soul of man. The latter, however, gets us into theology, and I would prefer to stay out of that — at least at this time. "What makes us tick as animals" is a more complicated question. There is involved not only our cerebral cortex but our adrenal cortices as well, to say nothing of the rest, both of our nervous systems and of our endocrine systems.

The great dynamic integrative mechanisms of the animal body are the nervous and circulatory systems and the endocrine system, which employs the circulation as its conveyor. These systems, which are integrated with one another, together play an indispensable role in the integration of the higher animal in its entirety.

But, one may ask, "What of the amoeba?" This lowly being seemingly gets on well without either an endocrine or a nervous system, yet it behaves as a beautifully integrated organism, better perhaps in some respects than man. Who, for example, ever heard of a schizophrenic amoeba? Does the amoeba make substances bearing any resemblance to hormones, or does it get on quite well without them? I suspect that it gets on without them, and that integration in single-celled existence is achieved through regulation of the rate of one enzyme system by the accumulated products of another enzyme system. We may call this enzymatic integration, or the primordial integration of the unicellular, and perhaps look upon it as the most primitive integrating mechanism of the multicellular. I will return to this interesting subject later.

When I was a medical student I read from cover to cover with rapt attention the work of Sherrington, then professor of physiology at Liverpool, entitled, *The Integrative Action of the Nervous System.*[1] It was his Silliman Lectures, delivered at Yale, and it represented the most authoritative work on the physiology of the nervous system of approximately half a century ago. Investigation since Sherrington's has added much to our understanding of the physiology of the nervous system, as, for example, the whole concept of the conditioned reflex of Pavlov,[2] the chemical mediation of nerve impulse, localization of function in the brain, etc., but I believe there is little, if anything, in Sherrington's conceptual scheme that requires retraction.

This work made a deep impression on me, and through the intervening years, as I have become increasingly interested in endocrinology, I have become more and more conscious of certain similarities between the functions of the nervous and the endocrine systems.

In both systems stimuli are received; signals are sent to distant end-organs which, upon receipt thereof, perform in turn the functions they have been evolved to perform. "The unit mechanism in integration by the nervous system," Sherrington tells us, "is the reflex," and in the reflex there are involved "at least three separable structures": receptors, conductors, and effectors. In the case of the nervous system, receptors are sense organs of one sort or another, conductors are neurones and synapses, and effectors are muscle or gland cells. The same terminology can be applied to the endocrine system. Receptors are the cells of endocrine glands or similar tissues, conductors are hormones, and effectors are the end-organs or targets upon which hormones specifically act. The simplest nervous reflex arc involves at least two neurones, but more complicated reactions require many more. So also in the endocrine system we often find hook-ups in which two or more hormones are involved. An important property of the nervous system also is that action on effectors may in some cases be excitatory, in others, inhibitory. The same is true of the endocrine system. Hormone *A*, for example, provokes the delivery of hormone *B*, but hormone *B* suppresses that of hormone *A*.

I do not wish to belabor the nervous-endocrine analogy unduly — it has, of course, but a limited application — nor do I wish to consider integration by the endocrine system as a thing apart. However, if the limitations of the analogy are recognized (and I hope, if not already obvious, they will emerge as I proceed), it will prove helpful in the development of a concept of total integration of the person, which is what, after all, concerns the physician.

The whole process of living, in its material realm, consists in everlastingly adjusting to environment. Adjustment includes not merely the erection of defenses against hurtful influences of environment, but also the alteration of environment by the organism to make it more suitable for the organism. Good adjustment is health; poor adjustment is illness. Successful adjustment is integration, unsuccessful is disintegration. When adjustment fails completely, life ceases or, if you prefer, death takes place. It is a case of "root, hog, or die." Frustration I should classify as a form of disintegration.

"In the multicellular animal," Sherrington tells us, "especially for those higher reactions which constitute its behaviour as a social unit in the natural economy, it is nervous reaction which par excellence integrates it, welds it together from its components, and constitutes it, from a mere collection of organs, an animal individual."

Sherrington admits that the animal possesses other integrating agencies, for example, "the mechanical combination of the unit cells of the body into a single mass." Also, he speaks of integration resulting from chemical agencies, as, for example, that resulting from the circulation of the blood. But extranervous phenomena were not his concern, and he said nothing further about them.

At approximately the same time that I was reading Sherrington I also had the good fortune to have as teacher of physiology Walter Bradford Cannon. At the time I was a medical student he was beginning his classic studies on the effect of the emotions on bodily processes and the development of his concept of homeostasis.[3] Unlike Sherrington, Cannon was concerned with both nervous and chemical, or endocrine, integrating mechanisms. He was less occupied with external behavior of the organism than with its methods of preserving the constancy of its internal environment, which Claude Bernard had recognized as the price of free and independent life. Therefore, he was more concerned with the vegetative, or autonomic, nervous system, which works inwardly on the viscera and governs internal environment, than with the central, which works outwardly; and of the two divisions of the autonomic nervous system he was more concerned with the sympathetic division, which discharges diffusely to the viscera, including blood vessels, than with the parasympathetic, which is focused more sharply on specific end-organs. In considering the integration of the nervous and the endocrine systems, one with the other, we shall have to take into account all divisions of the former, but in particular the sympathetic.

The endocrine system, like the nervous system, can be separated into certain divisions. On the one hand we have such organs as the adrenal medulla and the posterior pituitary (or neurohypophysis), which are clearly under direct neural control, and which even bear strong resemblances histologically to nervous tissue; while on the other we have the remaining, more obviously glandular, endocrine organs, which have not been proved to be under any direct neural control. I have been tempted to call the first category the para-endocrine system, to set it apart in our minds from all the rest of the endocrine system. The hormones of the para-endocrines — adrenalin and pituitrin — are quick acting and have widespread effects. They are secreted in response to stimuli reaching their parent cells directly over autonomic nervous pathways. The hormones of the remaining endocrines are more sharply focused on their targets. They are secreted in response to humoral, not neural, stimulation.

In the organizational pattern of the endocrine system in its present state of evolution in vertebrates, we find what I have called the para-endocrine system, occupying an intermediary position between the nervous and the endocrine systems proper. All impulses — at least so it appears — that pass from the nervous system to the endocrine — and we know beyond all possible doubt that such passages occur — must pass by way of the para-endocrines, reaching the para-endocrine glands neurally; they continue humorally (or, if you prefer, hormonally), seemingly only via the anterior lobe of the pituitary. From the anterior pituitary the organizational pattern may be described, in part at least, as a congeries of two-way hormonic pathways (or axes) radiating from the anterior lobe to one of the peripheral endocrine organs. In each case the two-way pathway is traversed on the outward journey by a tropic hormone of the anterior pituitary which stimulates the peripheral gland to make its hormone (or hormones), and on the return journey by the peripheral hormone, which in turn inhibits the pituitary with respect to that particular tropic function. This type of balanced reaction, which I shall call the axial principle, is semiautomatic, but not, as we shall see presently, completely independent unless it becomes so in disease. It may be looked upon as a functional unit of the endocrine system, analogous in some respects to the reflex arc of the nervous system. That the secretion by the pituitary of adenotropic hormones (that is, hormones whose targets are other endocrines) is controlled by the blood level of the hormones of the peripheral gland that is stimulated seems to be a fundamental law of the endocrine system. Knowledge of this law was first gained from the so-called castration phenomenon, that is to say, hypertrophy of the pituitary and increased secretion of the hormone tropic to the gonads that have been removed or destroyed. The phenomenon is well exemplified by the physiologic castration of the menopause, causing a great increase in secretion by the pituitary of gonadotropic hormone.

The axial principle is known to apply to the pituitary in its relation to the gonads, the thyroid, and the adrenal cortices. So far as I have discovered, there is no convincing evidence that the pituitary exercises any tropic action over the parathyroids or pancreatic islands. It also should be noted that the anterior pituitary makes certain hormones which act directly on nonendocrine endorgans, as, for example, prolactin and the growth hormone.

The ascendancy which the anterior pituitary has gained over the endocrine system may be likened to that of the cerebral cortex over the nervous system. As the cerebral cortex signals various parts of the soma over pathways of varying numbers of neurones, so does the pituitary at times send a hormone to impinge directly on an effector target — a melanophore, for example, or a mammary gland — while at others, the ultimate somatic target is reached via an intermediary endocrine, as pituitary to gonad to uterus, or pituitary to thyroid to muscle. In other words, the endocrines and their hormones may be coupled up as are neurones.

Whether there are important direct humoral balance relations between peripheral endocrines, one with another, not routed through or mediated by the anterior pituitary, I think is not known. Presumably there are what we may call nonspecific effects, as when an increasing output of thyroid hormone directly causes an increase in metabolic activity of other endocrines, along with the other cells of the body. For example, we have seen certain patients with far advanced athyreotic myxedema and evidences of reduced pituitary function in whom these evidences have vanished with restoration of the normal thyroid state. Premenopausal patients with severe myxedema often show oligomenorrhea and amenorrhea, and studies of the nature of these disorders have disclosed that the endometrium, via the ovary, may be under the influence of a diminshed pituitary secretion of follicle-stimulating hormone, and that there may be no evidence of any leutinizing hormone whatsoever. The normal functional gonadal hormonal balance is restored when thyroid is given to the patient. Some of our myxedematous patients have also shown some evidences of hypoadrenocorticism, and these abnormalities have also vanished when thyroid has been administered. It is a common observation of the gynecologists that fertility, either of the sterile male or female, can often be restored by dessicated thyroid, although the precise way in which this comes about is not yet clear. But action of this sort would not be in the same category as the specific balanced relations between the anterior lobe and the peripheral gland. The latter may be likened to a nervous reaction originating in and requiring the presence of the higher nerve centers, the former to reflex nervous phenomena which remain intact in the spinal animal. One pertinent fact is that in the case of the thyroid, at least, it can be shown that the gland's own hormone inhibits the gland directly. I have wondered if, phylogenetically speaking, this type of control of thyroid function represents a more ancient one than that mediated through the pituitary.

For a complete understanding of the modus operandi of the endocrine system as it exists in man and his nearer relatives in the animal scale, I have long believed that more knowledge of the evolutionary process is needed. From what primitive form did it evolve? Early in the multicellular story, enzymatic or, as I called it earlier, primordial integration may have sufficed, but only for very simple organisms living in very simple environments. As the struggle for survival has driven organisms into ever tougher environments, such superstructures as nervous and endocrine systems have of necessity been evolved in order to increase efficiency to the point where such environments can successfully be mastered.

In considering the nervous system, Sherrington discusses the nerve-cell network of the jellyfish Medusa. Here is a nervous system which receives stimuli and promotes coördinated movement of the whole organism, yet is without polarity or centralization. There is neither head nor tail to such a system, yet it adequately brings about adjustment of this particular organism to its particular environment. As we ascend the animal scale, the nervous system develops a linear and segmental arrangement — a head end gains dominance, culminating in the brain of man. Similarly, may not the endocrine system have begun without the segregation of endocrine tissues into specific glands, and, when glands were first evolved, may they not have been in more or less equal partnership, one with the others, without any one member being dominant in the sense that the anterior pituitary is now dominant? As a matter of fact, when I was a medical student that is about the way the endocrine system was visualized. We spoke of the ductless glands, not of the endocrine system, and we visualized them as operating pretty much as individuals. The present concept of what I have called the axial organization was quite unknown. The pituitary-thyroid axis, for example, did not enter our thinking on thyroid problems until after 1930, and then for some years we were rather inclined to conceive it as working pretty much as a self-regulating gadget, not much influenced from higher up.

Now, however, great interest is focused on the neuro-endocrine bridge, of which the anterior pituitary seems to be the keystone — particularly, on the question as to what is the approach to this bridge from the nervous system side. As yet the evidence bearing on this question is, on the whole, rather scant. To be sure, as early as 1914 Cannon showed that stimulation of the splanchnic nerves of the sympathetic nervous system caused a discharge of adrenalin from the adrenal medulla; also it seems likely, though the evidence is less clear cut, that the neurohypophysis is stimulated to secretory activity by nervous impulses reaching it via the stalk from the hypothalamus; but when we search for evidence of a direct pathway, either neural or humoral, between the neurohypophysis and the adenohypophysis, we end up in confusion. It is true that various forms of psychic activity are followed by alteration in function of the peripheral endocrines, but by what route is far from clear. Indeed, one cannot be sure that the intimate proximity of the neurohypophysis to the adenohypophysis, or of the adrenal medulla to the adrenal cortex, has any functional significance at all. It is possible that these juxtapositions are purely adventitious. Since evidence of direct secretory innervation of endocrines, except adrenal medulla and neurohypophysis, is unconvincing, we may postulate that for stimulation of the other glands a neurohumoral pathway is requisite. In the case of one of them — the adrenal cortex — the pathway, thanks largely to the work of Long and his collaborators, has been elucidated. With evidence now available, this pathway may be traced as follows:

Afferent impulses from the outside world and the muscular system impinge, through sense organs, upon the thalamus. Thence they are relayed to the higher levels of the brain, where they give rise to processes of cerebration, the emotional component of which activates the hypothalamus, which in turn excites the sympathetic nervous system, and with it, the adrenal medulla, with resulting discharge of adrenalin. Adrenalin, of course, has many and varied actions and a multiplicity of targets, among which, so Long's work suggests, is the adenohypophysis, which is stimulated to discharge adrenocorticotropic hormone or, as it is now universally called, ACTH. Thus one might refer to adrenalin, in this particular one of its roles, as a pituitary tropic hormone, or perhaps as adrenocorticotropic-tropic hormone. The next event in the chain of events is, of course, the stimulation of the adrenal cortex by ACTH to produce its own hormones, including the celebrated and glamorous cortisone, and these in turn, as their titer rises in the blood when they reach the pituitary, shut down the latter's output of ACTH, and thus the hormonic circle is completed.

Long and McDermott[4] claim a dual control of the secretion of ACTH by the pituitary. That which results directly from stimulation of anterior-lobe cells by adrenalin they call the "autonomic control"; that which results from a falling titer of cortical hormones in the blood they call the "metabolic." The concept is derived from the observation that in animals whose adrenal glands have been demedullated, and in animals in which destructive lesions have been produced in the thalamus and hypothalamus, the autonomic release of ACTH is abolished, whereas the metabolic response remains intact. It was further shown that homologous grafts of anterior-pituitary tissue to the anterior chamber of the eye retain their ability to secrete ACTH both spontaneously and in response to adrenalin. Moreover, it was found that adrenalin injected directly into the anterior chamber of the eye containing the transplant caused a response even when given in very minute doses, too small to have any direct systemic effect. In neither the adrenal demedullated animals nor those with diencephalic lesions could there be any reflex secretion of adrenalin, because in the former the gland which makes that hormone had been removed, and in the latter the reflex pathway had been interrupted. The transplanted anterior pituitary, however, subject only to hormonal stimulation, was able to respond either to administered adrenalin or spontaneously, under the control, presumably, of the blood titer of cortical hormones. These observations, which support a dual-control theory with respect to adrenocortical functions, interest me greatly, and I would dearly like to know whether similar dual control exists in the case of other glands. Indeed, is dual control a usual organizational pattern of the endocrine system? and, if so, what are the other tropic-tropic hormones involved? Is adrenaline tropic-tropic to all the peripheral glands, or are there others? If there are others, are they derived from the adrenal medulla, the posterior pituitary, or elsewhere? Indeed, we would like to know what role in the overall outflow from the nervous system to the endocrine system is played by the posterior pituitary. Certainly its hormone or hormones have widespread effects on blood sugar, on blood pressure, on the uterus, antidiuretic, etc., but are any of these mediated through the anterior-pituitary or peripheral endocrines? These are all fundamentally important questions, but I do not believe that, at the moment, any of them can be answered. The elucidation of the adrenocortical pathway got ahead of that of others, because of the great ease with which adrenocortical activity can be tested for by means of the eosinopenic response. No equally convenient and rapid assays for thyrotropic hormone and gonadotropic hormone have yet been devised. One can make eosinophil counts as often as one likes; there is nothing to parallel this for the other tropic hormones. In the case of the thyroid there is some pertinent evidence, but it is hardly conclusive. Salter, for example, cited evidence that the blood iodine level rises after the administration of adrenalin, which fact would at least be consistent with a thyrotropic-tropic action of adrenalin, and Uotila[5] has obtained results supporting a dual control for thyrotropic activity of the anterior lobe analogous to Long's for adrenocorticotropic. Uotila found that hyperplasia of the thyroid which follows exposure to cold fails to take place if the pituitary stalk is cut, but that control of thyrotropic activity is effected by blood thyroxine level whether the stalk is cut or not.

I suppose by now the reader will feel entitled to an apology for terminology. Para-endocrine — that is to say, beside the endocrine — seems to me fair enough, but what of tropic-tropic? Can he bear with that? One may say, why tropic at all — why not trophic? Both these suffixes are in common use. What do they signify? Tropic is derived from τροπή, meaning turn — perhaps, turn toward. Trophic, from τροφικός, clearly carries the implication of something having to do with nutrition. It seems to me that to imply a nutritional quality to the impingement of a pituitary hormone upon its end-organ is to be more specific than existing knowledge justifies. "Tropic," meaning turned toward, or "aimed at," commits us to far less and therefore, in our ignorance, seems a more suitable term. Thyrotropic can be taken to mean aimed at the thyroid. Of course all hormones are aimed at some target; therefore, one might say all are tropic, and that the suffix is superfluous. It is convenient, however, when the target of one hormone when hit discharges another, to use the suffix tropic to define the former. Also, when a target is hit by a hormone and thereupon discharges a second hormone which hits a second target which discharges a third hormone, it seems to me reasonable to apply to the first hormone of the series the term tropic-tropic.

And this discussion brings me to the subject of targets or end-organs, a little-known area of endocrine physiology, but quite as essential to a comprehensive understanding of the workings of the endocrine system as is a knowledge of the synapse or the myoneural junction to an understanding of the nervous system. My own work has dealt with the thyroid, therefore I will discuss the action of the thyrotropic and thyroid hormones upon their targets by way of illustration.

The target of the thyrotropic hormone is the parenchyma of the thyroid gland. What happens when this hormone hits this target? There is available a certain amount of evidence bearing on this question, and it will be easiest to interpret it if we think in terms of the known functions of the thyroid gland. These all have to do with the manufacture of its hormone and may be identified as follows:

1. A mechanism for trapping iodide from the blood stream.
2. Synthesis of thyroxine. This involves iodination of tyrosine

to diiodotryosine and the coupling of two molecules of the latter to form thyroxine, all these reactions taking place within the chain molecule of thyroid protein — thyroglobulin.

3. Storage of hormone as thyroglobulin within the thyroid follicles.

4. Discharge of hormone to the body.

Study of the action of thyrotropic hormone (TTH) on these functions has been facilitated by the fact that we now have drugs capable of divorcing these several thyroid functions. Potassium sulfocyanate, for example, blocks the trapping mechanism. So do perchlorate and certain other anions. Thiouracil and its relations, on the other hand block the synthetic mechanism. Thyrotropic hormone probably promotes all the functions of the thyroid but, when part is blocked, will accelerate the unblocked. Thus the gland blocked with thiouracil will still trap iodine when TTH is administered. It will also liberate hormone, which, in view of the fact that the synthetic mechanism is blocked, must mean that TTH promotes the breakdown of stored thyroglobulin. The releasing of hormone may be the earliest effect of TTH on the thyroid. The work of De Robertis[6] suggests that it is due to almost immediate activation of the proteolytic enzyme system of the thyroid, which brings about a reduction in the molecular size of stored protein and permits thyroxine-containing fractions to escape to the circulation. Hypertrophy and hyperplasia of thyroid parenchyma then follow with increased trapping of iodine and, finally, 48 hours or more after injection of TTH, increased synthesis of hormone.

In brief, these are the things TTH does to the thyroid gland. Now the question becomes, What does the thyroid do to TTH in the process? Rawson[7] and his collaborators have shown that when TTH acts on the thyroid it disappears. This disappearance, however, is not due to destruction, because hormonic activity can be restored by heat or by certain mild reducing agents. The hormone is inactivated only, and remains capable of reactivation.

It can be found in the urine in its inactivated form and, under certain circumstances, also in its active form.

The question of whether TTH has any specific targets, or end-organs, other than the thyroid cells, is important. When Rawson studied inactivation of TTH by thyroid tissue, he also made observations on other tissues, and found that both lymph-node tissue and thymus caused partial inactivation. Adrenal, kidney, ovary, pancreas, parathyroid, testis, spleen, and stomach mucosa caused none. Interpretation of these findings is not possible. All that can be said is that thymus and lymph-node tissue do something to TTH. What, if anything, TTH does to them is not known. However, the suggestion is strong that these tissues are in some way targets for TTH. Somewhat stronger evidence connects TTH with the orbits. For some years now this hormone has been believed connected in some way with the ophthalmopathy of Graves's disease. At least it has been found experimentally that anterior-pituitary extracts rich in thyrotropic principle cause marked exophthalmos in animals. This is accompanied in the orbit by edema and the laying down of connective-tissue cellular elements, lymphocytes, macrophages, and fibroblasts. This is a picture similar to that seen in humans with Graves's disease.

The other hormone involved in the pituitary-thyroid axis is thyroid hormone. How does that one impinge on its end-organs; also, what are its end-organs? Presumably all cells in the body are targets or end-organs to the thyroid hormone, and its action on them is to stimulate their metabolic processes. This is a well-known fact. However, in two special instances thyroid hormone inhibits its end-organs. As already mentioned, it inhibits the anterior pituitary in its thyrotropic function, and it inhibits the thyroid gland itself. When we come to the problem of the mechanism whereby the thyroid hormone exerts its action on its target we can find very little pertinent information. Presumably, thyroxine diffuses into the cell; at least, Professor Fritz Lipmann informs me that he finds it within cells in about the same concentration as in the serum, and distributed fairly evenly through-out the various elements of the cell. But how it exerts its action on the enzyme systems of the cell, and what happens to it in the process, remain to be elucidated.

Let us now turn again to the working of the endocrine system as a whole. One way of studying the nature of an integrating mechanism is to throw it out of gear at various points and ob-serve what then happens. In the case of the endocrine system we can ablate portions of the system; we can administer hormones and, quite as important, we can investigate nature's endocrine disintegrations, namely, endocrine disease. It was from the last-mentioned method, of course, that the first knowledge of the endocrine system was obtained.

There was a time when it was believed that by removing a single endocrine gland, or by giving a single pure hormone, one could isolate the action of one gland from the rest. But this is obviously not so. In a system made of infinitely interrelated mechanisms, as is the animal body, or at least the bodies of higher animals, one cannot alter any one part of the mechanism without altering the rest, for the rest must adjust to the disturbed part in order that commotion in the whole be kept at a minimum. Those physicians and surgeons who deal with a very restricted part of the body would do well from time to time to ponder these truths.

I will mention a few items that may illustrate what I mean. Aside from Addison's early recognition of the consequence of destruction of the adrenals, the important early endocrinology had to do with the thyroid. The connection of the thyroid with the clinical picture of myxedema, the discovery that feeding thy-roid would remove this picture, seemed to tell most, or all, of the story about this particular endocrine organ. The role of the pituitary in thyroid function was not at all suspected, even though as early as 1851 a French physician, Nièpce, had made the important observation that the pituitary is hypertrophied in cretins. The significance of Nièpce's work was not apparent until years after, when TTH had made its appearance on the medical scene.

It was in 1889 that von Mering and Minkowski showed that pancreatectomy caused diabetes mellitus in dogs. In 1922 Banting and Best obtained insulin from the pancreas, which relieved it. The situation in diabetes, however, is not as simple as that of the thyroid and myxedema; in fact, it is very complicated. In 1931 Houssay and Biasotti[8] found that hypophysectomy prevents or ameliorates the diabetes caused by pancreatectomy, and from this emerged the concept of a diabetogenic hormone of the anterior pituitary which directly antagonizes insulin. In 1935 Long and Lukens[9] brought the adrenal cortex into the picture by discovering that adrenalectomy also ameliorates pancreatic diabetes. The hormone of the adrenal cortex of the 11-oxysteroid type, popularly known as cortisone, inhibits the oxidation of carbohydrate and, so Ingle has shown, causes violent aggravation of pancreatic diabetes and great resistance to insulin. The amelioration of pancreatic diabetes following adrenalectomy is believed to be due to the removal from the situation of the cortical diabetogenic hormone, cortisone. The diabetes of Cushing's syndrome is the result of the excessive production of diabetogenic cortisone by this hyperfunctioning cortex. It is insulin-resistant.

Thus at least three endocrines are brought into the diabetes picture, and we can bring in a fourth if we wish, namely, the thyroid. It has long been known that giving thyroid aggravates diabetes mellitus, and that when a diabetic person develops myxedema the diabetes is ameliorated. I have long supposed that these facts were to be explained on the basis of increased general (including carbohydrate) metabolism, by the thyroid hormone. Diabetes is aggravated by thyroid because the higher metabolism imposes a greater burden on the glucose-burning mechanism, and removal of the thyroid gland diminishes it. But the thyroid may also play a more complex role. There is some evidence that hyperthyroidism also occasions hyperadrenocorticism. By what mechanism I do not know. The point is, however, that in addition to putting an extra strain on the sugar mechanism directly, hyperthyroidism may also call forth an increased discharge of diabetogenic cortical hormone. Houssay has found that giving thyroid to partially pancreatectomized dogs produces a type of diabetes indistinguishable from the usual form of pancreatic diabetes. When thyroid is withdrawn the diabetes disappears. He calls this "thyroid diabetes." If thyroid is continued long enough, an irreversible change may take place and a permanent diabetes result. This he calls "metathyroid diabetes."

The endocrine system is largely concerned in the now famous alarm reaction or adaptation syndrome of Selye.[10] This investigator was bright enough to recognize that nearly any variety of violence or noxious stimulus, if sufficiently strong, sets off a chain reaction in the vertebrate animal which seemingly, at least in the healthy animal, is useful in preparing it to cope with the disturbing situation. In the diseased subject — the diabetic, for example, or the thyrotoxic — the alarm reaction may be highly injurious or even fatal by adding the extra burden of an adrenocortical diabetes to the preëxisting pancreatic or thyroid diabetes, thus throwing the patient in the former case into diabetic acidosis and coma, and in the latter, into thyrotoxic crisis or so-called thyroid storm. Under such circumstances we may say that the endocrine integrating mechanism does not integrate — instead, it disintegrates the organism. Dr. Janet W. McArthur has made very extensive metabolic studies on a diabetic patient in the research ward of the Massachusetts General Hospital, and finds that even the withholding of insulin provokes an alarm reaction, with increased output of cortical hormones.

If, as the examples I have cited would seem to indicate, the endocrine glands are normally all in balance one with another, the effect of removing a part of them, or of giving an excess of the hormones of any of them, will obviously unbalance the system or throw it out of gear. I have wondered for many years, however, what would happen if the entire endocrine system could be ablated. This question came to my mind because of Cannon's experiments on the total ablation of the sympathico-adrenal system. Cats so operated on continued to live without apparent difficulty in the sheltered environment of the laboratory, but there were many adjustments they were quite unable to make, and they were totally unable to cope with the tough type of world in which a cat normally has to make its way. To conquer such an environment, the superstructure of a sympathetic nervous system is requisite.

And in the case of hormones, Long has made the point that they "do not initiate new patterns of cellular function; these are in the birthright of the cells themselves. All that any hormone does is either to facilitate or inhibit certain types of chemical transformation within the cells." If this concept is correct, one might speculate that as Cannon's cats got on in a limited way without their sympathetic nervous systems, so might animals deprived of their endocrine system make a shift to carry on the adaptive process in a limited way in a sheltered environment. But be that as it may, it is certain that, for normal living by the higher animal, an intact endocrine system is as requisite as an intact nervous system.

I would like to conclude with some comments on the present all-prevailing ACTH-cortisone furor. On all sides the time-honored principle of substitution therapy is being violated. In a subject whose thyroid is atrophic, we give a quantity of thyroid hormone which presumably approximates what his own thyroid gland would be making if it were capable of normal function. So doing restores the subject to a state approaching that of complete health. This is substitution therapy. When we give insulin in pancreatic diabetes we are also providing substitution therapy, although in this case, because the hormone is fast acting instead of slow like thyroid, it is more difficult to adjust the dose with great nicety to the precise need of the organism. Thyroid hormone provides specific substitution therapy only for athyreosis or myxedema, as it is usually called. Insulin provides it only for pancreatic diabetes. When large doses of cortisone (or ACTH to stimulate the secretion of cortisone) are given in a host of diseases, it is certainly not substitution therapy in the usual meaning of the word. Such therapy is based on a totally different principle. It is not a matter of supplying in physiologic amounts a hormone that is lacking; it is rather one of giving a great excess of a hormone in the hope of thus neutralizing some injurious process which is causing the malady. We can quite properly regard myxedema as a deficiency disease — deficiency of thyroid hormone — but assuredly we cannot consider rheumatoid arthritis, asthma, lymphoma, or any other of the diseases which have been reported to be benefited by these new hormones, as in any similar sense diseases simply due to deficiency of these hormones.

One can perhaps for a time neutralize the inroads of a morbid process by giving an excess of a hormone, as one can with a drug, but in so doing one cannot be said to have rebuilt a normal status, in the sense that one does by giving thyroid in myxedema. If a therapy produces a permanent change in a subject, then the subject must effect an adjustment to the therapy.

The situation may be likened to that in which one tries to bring to even keel a boat with a list to starboard by putting a load to port. Perhaps the boat *is* righted, but the original situation has not been restored. The boat is more heavily laden than it was and, if the load imposed is too heavy, the boat may sink!

What has happened in the few years since the nonphysiologic use of ACTH and cortisone has been in vogue is that an increasing number of untoward side effects have been encountered. As the use of these hormones is extended, we shall see still more. According to the philosophy I have been trying to enunciate, such therapy, although productive of immediate symptomatic benefit, must be looked upon as, in its fundamental nature, disintegrating, and its use should be governed with that concept in mind. I close with that warning.

2 The thyroid hormone

In any consideration of the function of the thyroid gland, one is concerned largely with the thyroid hormone and with the thyrotropic hormone of the pituitary. The latter may conveniently be called thyrotropin. Our knowledge of these hormones is as yet fragmentary. We do know that together they form a balanced system, being reciprocally excitatory and inhibitory, the pituitary stimulating the thyroid and the thyroid inhibiting the pituitary, with respect to thyrotropic action — an example, to use present jargon, of the feedback principle.

The type of knowledge which we now possess of these two hormones is different. Thanks chiefly to the masterly work of Sir Charles R. Harington[1, 2] for example, we know a great deal of the biosynthesis of thyroxine. Of the mechanism by which thyroid hormone affects its targets, however, we know distressingly little. In the case of thyrotropin, the work of Rawson[3, 4] and of others has given us some insight into the manner in which this hormone affects targets, but of its biosynthesis, or even of the rate of its production, we know nothing. The gaps in our knowledge are due, in part at least, to lack of certain technical approaches.

I would like first to set a background for a discussion of the thyroid hormone by recalling a few salient items of medical history. It is of interest that the first fundamental knowledge of the thyroid was gained largely by clinicians. Thus as early as 1820 Coindet in Switzerland showed that giving iodine relieved certain types of goiter, and in 1850 Curling in England found complete atrophy of the thyroid in sporadic cretins. The physiologist Schiff of Geneva in 1859 obtained hypothyroid manifestations in animals by thyroidectomy, but in 1874 Gull in England, although he gave an excellent clinical description of spontaneous myxedema in humans, stated that he was "not able to give any explanation of the cause." However, in 1883 the surgeon Kocher of Bern found that total thyroidectomy in humans produced the picture of Gull's disease. Finally substitution therapy for athyreosis emerged from the work of Bettencourt and Serrano in 1890 in France, and of Murray and of Fenwick in England, both of whom published in 1891. It was from such observations, as well as those of others, that the concept of a hormone peculiar to the thyroid gland took its origin.[5]

This concept having been formed, the biochemists set to work to isolate an active principle. Baumann in Germany in 1896 discovered that iodine is a normal constituent of the thyroid, and by acid hydrolysis of the gland's proteins he separated a small fraction containing about 10 per cent of iodine, which he called iodothyrin. This substance administered to patients with hypothyroidism was found to possess physiologic properties like those of whole thyroid gland.

In 1911 Oswald isolated from the thyroid the iodine-bearing amino acid diiodotyrosine. This, however, possesses no physiologic activity. The most important event following Baumann's discovery of iodine in the thyroid was the isolation from the gland by Kendall in 1915 in pure crystalline form the amino acid thyroxine, which he found to possess the full physiologic activity of whole thyroid substance, and which he showed contains 60 per cent by weight of iodine.

The next crucial observations on the biochemistry of the thyroid hormone came in 1926 when Harington[6] identified the structural formula of thyroxine as a hydroxyphenylether of tyrosine containing four atoms of iodine in the 3, 5, 3', 5' position, and the following year when Harington and Barger achieved its synthesis.[7]

Harington and Barger synthesized thyroxine in the laboratory. It had never been done there before. But nature must have been biosynthesizing thyroxine in the bodies of animals for aeons, although we do not know just how far back in the evolutionary scale the process began. Harington and Barger's synthesis was accomplished by a complicated series of chemical reactions involving, altogether, eight different steps, but their work disclosed that nature effects her biosynthesis by iodinating tyrosine to diiodotyrosine, and then by coupling two molecules of diiodotyrosine, with the loss of one side chain, to form one molecule of thyroxine.

The next bit of background that we need for what follows is that in the organism this synthesis seems to take place only within the matrix of a protein molecule. When the process occurs in the thyroid, the protein matrix is thyroglobulin. Whether there is any true *in vivo* extrathyroidal biosynthesis of thyroid hormone is a disputed question. If there is any it must be insignificant in amount. *In vitro*, however, a variety of proteins may be exposed to elemental iodine, and if the pH is right, iodination of protein will occur and thyroidlike physiologic activity will be acquired. This has been shown to be due to actual formation of thyroxine.

Until very recently the general belief had been that thyroxine is itself the thyroid hormone. All variations made in the thyroxine molecule had reduced or abolished its physiologic activity. Until about a year ago the only iodine-bearing amino acids found in the thyroid had been moniodotyrosine, diiodotyrosine, and tetraiodothyronine or thyroxine. Then, however, Gross and Pitt-Rivers[8] in Harington's laboratory discovered by means of paper chromatography traces of a fourth substance in this series, namely, triiodothyronine. They were able to make physiologic tests with this material, and found that not only did it possess full thyroxinelike activity, but it had, weight for weight, several times the potency.

This discovery was a bombshell to theoretical thyroidology. I will return to its significance a little later.

I must add one final touch to the background. Then I will try to paint a foreground. The point is that the thyroid gland does not operate in glorious isolation. It is but a member of a co-ordinated system of endocrine organs functionally dependent on the nervous system, which two systems together constitute the chief integrating mechanism of the higher animal organism.

The type of hormonal balance which I have already mentioned as existing between the pituitary and the thyroid, exists also between the pituitary and the gonad, and the adrenal cortex. Such "axes," as Salter[9] has called them, may exist in the case of other endocrines. They constitute self-regulating mechanisms in which each of two glands involved is controlled through the blood level of the hormone of the other, and to some extent by that of its own.

When I began my career in medicine at the end of the first decade of the century, the tropic hormone of the pituitary had not been recognized as such. It was not until the late twenties that such terms as "thyroid stimulator" appeared, and the first use of "thyreotropic" that I am aware of is that of Crew and Wiesner in 1930.[10] Yet facts were available a century ago from which the existence of a pituitary thyrotropic principle could have been deduced. I refer to the fundamentally significant discovery of the French physician Nièpce,[11] who in 1851 showed that the pituitary is characteristically enlarged in cretins. He had five autopsies; in each case the pituitary was hypertrophic. It is easy enough now to recognize the great importance of Nièpce's observation, but in the century which has elapsed since it was made it has attracted but scanty attention. I would like to put in a plug for Nièpce.

I have called the pituitary-thyroid axis self-regulating, and so it is from the peripheral side. That is to say, it will presumably supply thyroid hormone to the body in relation to the use of that hormone by the body, the objective of the mechanism being the maintenance of a relatively constant level of thyroid hormone in the blood — an example, I should say, of what Cannon called homeostasis.

A similar situation has been shown, chiefly by the work of C. N. H. Long[12] and his collaborators, to exist in the case of the adrenal cortex. Control of cortical hormone output through blood level of the hormone acting on the anterior pituitary, Long calls the "metabolic" control. However, he has further shown that there is another control mechanism which consists in the activation of the anterior pituitary to put out ACTH, by adrenalin. This he calls the "autonomic" control. It may be considered a method of meeting emergencies. Whether there is an analogous "autonomic" control of thyroid function has not been established, but there are some reasons to believe that there is.

With this brief sketch of how the thyroid works in relation to the rest of the body, let us now turn to its intrinsic activities. These may be identified as being sequentially (1) trapping of iodide, (2) biosynthesis of hormone, (3) storage of hormone as thyroglobulin in the thyroid follicle, (4) discharge of hormone to the circulation, (5) transport to targets, (6) action upon targets, (7) final fate of the hormone. I will examine certain aspects of some of these.

The thyroid gland is utterly unique in that for the manufacture of its hormone it requires an element — iodine — not used specifically by any other tissue. Without an adequate supply of iodine it cannot perform its function, namely, that of maintaining the metabolic rate of the body. It is not surprising, therefore, to find that it possesses a special mechanism for trapping iodide from the blood flowing through it.

When inorganic iodine is ingested and absorbed it circulates through the body as iodide. Like chloride, it is distributed chiefly in the extracellular fluid. When it reaches the thyroid it is specifically collected and concentrated. Thus the thyroid of the normal rat has been shown to concentrate ionic iodide to 20 times the concentration in the blood, and thyroids made hyperplastic with either thyrotropin or thiouracil can concentrate iodide up to 250 times the blood concentration. From the time that iodide reaches the blood stream from without, the thyroid and the kidney, which excretes it, are in competition for it.

It is customary in thinking about thyroidal iodine, to distinguish between an inorganic fraction and an organically bound fraction. The former is freely dialyzable, the latter is nondialyzable; the former can be discharged from the gland by an excess of thiocyanate ion, the latter cannot. Organically bound iodine in the thyroid is undoubtedly incorporated in the molecules of the iodine-bearing amino acids, which have been shown to be constantly present in the gland. It is in firm chemical combination. The achievement of this chemical union is an essential part of the process of hormone biosynthesis. It can be blocked by drugs of the thiouracil type. The amazing thing, however, is that the gland, totally blocked in its synthetic activity by such a drug, still traps inorganic iodide as well as ever. The trapping mechanism can be divorced from the biosynthetic. The question is — what is its nature?

There are, of course, several levels at which the answer to such a question can be sought — those, for example, of naturally occurring disease, *in vivo* experiments on animals, at the *in vitro* levels of intact living tissue (slices of thyroid), and finally of homogenates of one sort or another made from thyroid tissue. I will cite first some evidence gained from patients.

Stanbury and Hedge in our clinic were able to make radioiodine studies on three out of four goiterous cretins from a single family, and on one normal sibling; also on a single similar case from an unrelated family. These patients were sporadic, not endemic, cretins. Ordinarily sporadic cretins do not have goiters. In endemic cretins the goiter is a result of iodine want. When sporadic cretins have goiters some cause other than extrinsic iodine want must be looked for. Radioiodine tracer studies disclosed that the thyroid glands of the three cretins, and also of the normal sibling, all were able to accumulate iodide. On the

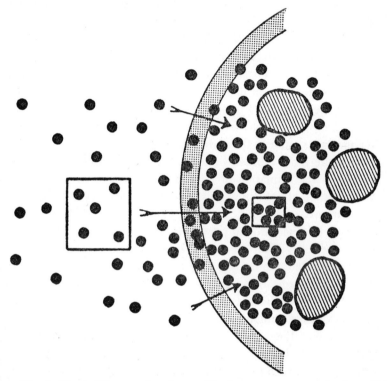

Fig. 1. The iodide trap, first theory. The long curve represents the wall of a thyroid cell, the black dots represent iodide ions, and the three larger ovoid symbols represent protein molecules. According to this theory, iodide is increted into the thyroid cell to reach a higher concentration than in the extracellular fluid.

administration of potassium thiocyanate the thyroids of the cretins promptly discharged their iodide, whereas that of the normal sibling retained it. It was concluded that, whereas the cretinous members of the family were able to trap iodide in their thyroids in a normal manner, for some reason not known, perhaps an inherited imperfection in the iodinating enzyme system, they were unable to iodinate the tyrosine nucleus and so could make no hormone. Their goiters, which anatomically were no different from those found in severe endemic areas, were the expression of an intrinsic unavailability of iodine.

The ease with which thiocyanate liberates or displaces iodide, or, to put it another way, the high degree of reversibility of iodide collection *in vivo*, suggests that its attachment in the thyroid must be very labile in nature. Two possible explanations of this process occur to one. First, as shown in Fig. 1, the thyroid cells may selectively increte iodide against a concentration gradient in a manner similar to the reabsorption process carried out by the cells of the renal tubules, or to that of the gastric mucosa with respect to the formation of hydrochloric acid, or to that of the concentration of potassium and magnesium by all cells. A second, and perhaps more likely, explanation is that iodide is simply adsorbed by some protein present in the thyroid cells which possesses a specific affinity for the iodide ion, as shown in Fig. 2. If one could isolate the trapping mechanism and determine whether it requires energy, one might be able to choose between these two possibilities. The first would require energy, the second might not. However, I do not know how this could be accomplished.

The observations on the goiterous cretins led to studies now in progress at the *in vitro* level by Wyngaarden, Stanbury, and Du Toit,[13] in which use is made of certain acellular homogenates of thyroid tissue. Two types of material are being investigated — the thyroids of normal rats and rat thyroids depleted of iodine. For control purposes other tissues than thyroid have been used — striated muscle, spleen, liver, kidney, and blood serum.

Making use of I^{131} (radioactively labeled iodine) the trapping of iodide across a cellophane membrane by these materials has been investigated. Dialysis is carried out for various periods of time up to 72 hours, at varying temperatures from $1°C$ upward.

By this method it has been found that the homogenates of thyroid, whether normal or depleted of iodine, consistently bind iodide. The depleted homogenate binds iodide in direct proportion to the concentration of iodide in the dialysate until a binding

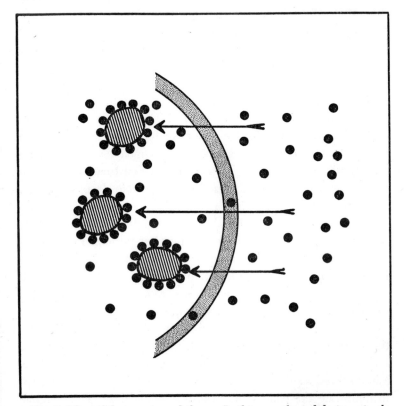

Fig. 2. The iodide trap, second theory. In this case the iodide ions simply diffuse into the thyroid cell and become adsorbed on protein.

of one-tenth gamma of iodide per milligram of thyroid protein has been reached. The total binding of iodide by this homogenate exceeds its original concentration of iodide by a factor of two or more.

The other tissues studied bound only insignificant amounts of iodide, with the single exception of blood serum, which, when highly diluted, binds iodide two-thirds as well as thyroid. However, with serum on one side of the membrane and thyroid homogenate on the other, the two being at nearly the same concentration of protein, the thyroid preparation will bind iodide from the serum. By means of chromatography it has been possible to show that much of the iodide collected by the thyroid homogenate is present in the form of inorganic iodide. Another experiment was designed to discover whether the collection of iodide by thyroid homogenates is reversible, as was that by the thyroid glands of Stanbury and Hedge's cretins. When exposed first to appropriate concentrations of thiocyanate, homogenates became unable to collect iodide. However, homogenates that had already collected iodide did not release it when treated with thiocyanate, nor could it be dialyzed off from them. In other words, in the case of this *in vitro* iodide collection, reversibility has not been demonstrated. The lack of reversibility of iodide collection by the homogenate is puzzling, but perhaps in some respects analogous to the binding of iron by serum. If the process is irreversible, iodide should not be present as such, and yet it is so present. This leaves us with a paradox. The work is being continued in the hope of clarifying it.

Another approach to the trapping problem has been through the study of the thiocyanate effect. Wyngaarden, Stanbury, and Rapp[14] have found that, mole for mole, iodide and thiocyanate, administered to the animal, are approximately equally effective in inhibiting the concentration of a labeling dose of radioactive iodine by the gland blocked with a thiouracil-like drug, or, to put it another way, radioiodide occupying the iodide space of the gland can be discharged by equimolecular doses of either iodide or thiocyanate. On the other hand, it was found, using material labeled with S^{35}, that the blocked gland is able to concentrate the S^{35} of labeled thiocyanate ion only to about ten times the serum concentration, whereas similar glands can achieve a concentration ratio for iodide 100 times that of serum, or better. The interesting paradox here is that, whereas the gland develops a much smaller concentration ratio for the S^{35} of labeled thiocyanate than for iodide, molar equivalent doses of the two have the same effect on the uptake of radioactive iodine given simultaneously.

Another development from our laboratory has been the use of perchlorate ion in experiments precisely similar to those with thiocyanate. Perchlorate is about ten times as effective as thiocyanate in preventing the accumulation of I^{131} by the thyroid. It is not yet known whether perchlorate is actually selectively concentrated by the gland as is thiocyanate.

Following the trapping of iodide, the next step in the process which leads to the elaboration of thyroid hormone is the oxidizing of trapped iodide to iodine. There is no free iodine to be found in the gland so that we must assume that, on the oxidation of iodide, iodine is immediately combined with tyrosine to form first monoiodotyrosine and then diiodotyrosine. In contrast to the trapping of iodide, which may require no energy, the oxidation of iodide to iodine requires high energy. A peroxidase system is the only one known with high enough redox potential to promote this reaction, and Dempsey[15] and others have found peroxidase in the thyroid.

The next step, namely, the conversion of diiodotyrosine to thyroxine, requires less energy than the preceding, but nevertheless is believed also to be an enzymatically promoted reaction.

The final event, that is to say, the delivery of thyroglobulin containing thyroxine into the follicles, Salter described almost lyrically as follows: "The parenchymal cells spew their protoplasm out into the follicle much as lacteal (mammary) cells produce milk globules in the lactating breast" — perhaps a good analogy. "It is possible, therefore, that the manufacture of hormone can occur within the follicle proper, at least in part, by virtue of the naked protoplasm extruded from the parenchymal cells."

What determines the rate of release of hormone from the gland? This is important, for the rate of release determines the setting of the metabolic rate of the organism. It is well known that removal of the adenohypophysis is followed by atrophy of the thyroid and failure of hormone release. Conversely, administration of thyrotropin will maintain the structure and function of the thyroid in the hypophysectomized animal. It has not been clear, however, whether thyrotropin stimulates all phases of thyroid activity, or that this is seemingly so only because increased activity of one phase is followed *pari passu* by an increase in the next succeeding phase.

In an attempt to pinpoint the site of action of thyrotropin Goldsmith, Stanbury and Brownell [16] measured the release rate of radioiodine in thyroids of thyrotoxic subjects given an effective antithyroid drug, 1-methyl-2-mercaptoimidazole. When the release curve, which is a straight line when plotted logarithmically, was well established, a series of injections of thyrotropin was given. Immediately there was a sharp increase in the release rate. Since the factor of hormone synthesis was controlled by the blocking agent, the conclusion reached was that thyrotropin causes the release of hormone independently of its effects on trapping and synthesis. Whether there are other factors controlling the release rate remains for further investigation.

Iodide is also involved in the secretion process. This was first pointed out by Means and Lerman[17] when they found that the time course of fall in basal metabolic rate is the same in the patient with Graves's disease who is treated with potassium iodide as it is when a total thyroidectomy is performed, or when a source of exogenous thyroid is withdrawn. The same effect of iodide has been demonstrated by Purves in New Zealand and by Goldsmith in Cincinnati when they found that therapeutic administration of potassium iodide inhibits the release of labeled hormone from the gland.

At this point it is appropriate to speculate about the significance of the structure of thyroxine. Although, as previously said, there is reason to believe that this substance is synthesized within the thyroglobulin molecule, that it is stored in the follicles in chemical combination with thyroglobulin, that it is released from the thyroid by the enzymatic breakdown of thyroglobulin, and that it is transported in the blood stream in association with plasma proteins, nevertheless it seems now safe to assert that thyroxine itself either *is* the thyroid hormone, or at least the business part of it, the warhead, so to speak, of the torpedo! It is reasonable to liken it to a torpedo, for after all it is aimed at a target! Possibly as it strikes the target it is converted into triiodothyronine.

The thyroxine molecule we may well regard as a remarkable structure. Take a look at it:

$$HO \overbrace{\underbrace{\bigcirc}_{I}}^{I} - O - \overbrace{\underbrace{\bigcirc}_{I}}^{I} CH_2CHNH_2COOH.$$

It is the only known hormone which is an amino acid, and, according to Harington, it is the only known naturally occurring product containing a diphenylether linkage.

Without an adequate supply of this potent compound normal life cannot go on, at least at the vertebrate level. It has no naturally occurring close relative that we know of except Triiodothyronine — no great flock of related substances all having hormonic activity, as is the case with the steroids.

Let us scrutinize its architecture and see what inferences can be drawn as to why it is built the way it is. What are the functions of its several parts? To what does it owe its unique catalytic capacity? I well remember a lecture by Barger given in Boston in 1928. "It's as though," said he, "one tadpole had swallowed the tail of another," and the eyes of the tadpoles are in positions corresponding to the I's of the molecule! We would like to know the function of its various components or radicals, as, for example, the iodine atoms, the diphenyl arrangement, the coupling of the two benzene rings, the side chain (or tail, keeping the tadpole in mind), and the hydroxyl group at the "anterior" end.

A method of approaching this question is by the bioassay of analogues of thyroxine on suitable test objects and the comparison of the result obtained, as quantitatively as may be, with that obtained in the case of thyroxine itself. The effect on physiologic response of various departures in molecular structure can thus be identified. As a matter of fact, Harington and his co-workers started using this approach shortly after the synthesis of thyroxine, and during the intervening years a number of other investigators,[18] including ourselves, have done likewise. The test objects have included normal and thyroidectomized animals in which the effect on metabolic rate is determined before and after the material is given, and tadpoles in which the effect on metamorphosis is quantitated. In our own work, which started with Salter's return from Harington's laboratory in the autumn of 1929 with a bottle of thyroxine polypeptide in his pocket, and which has continued ever since, we have always made use of human beings suffering from spontaneous myxedema as our test objects.

The objective has been to test every analogue of thyroxine that we could lay our hands on. Most of them were supplied to us by Harington. The work started off under the direct charge of Salter and Lerman, and after Salter's going to Yale in 1941, under that of Lerman.

It may be said at once that every variant from the thyroxine molecule, except triiodothyronine, that has been assayed has shown less physiologic activity than the naturally occurring substance. In other words, any alteration that has been made in molecular structure has yielded a substance of diminished (or absent) physiological activity.

In the first place there is the matter of optical activity. Naturally occurring thyroxine is laevorotatory. When one gives parenterally pure dextrorotatory thyroxine, it produces a response about one-tenth that of pure laevorotatory in magnitude.

In our studies of thyroxine analogues conducted on patients with myxedema, we have always related the physiologic action (effect on basal metabolic rate) of the substance being tested to that of pure laevorotatory thyroxine.

First we may consider the role of the diphenyl skeleton. For example, does diiodotyrosine,

$$HO \overline{\underset{I}{\overset{I}{\bigcirc}}} CH_2CHNH_2COOH,$$

the building block from which thyroxine is made, have any physiologic activity? It is possible, but it is of a very low order of magnitude, about 0.005 percent that of l-thyroxine. All of the diphenyl compounds tested, provided they had any halogens, had far greater activity than diiodotyrosine. Thyronine with no halogens is inert, or nearly so.

A compound like thyroxine, but with only two iodines, 3–5 diiodothyronine,

$$HO \overline{\bigcirc} - O - \overline{\underset{I}{\overset{I}{\bigcirc}}} CH_2CHNH_2COOH,$$

was 1.3 percent as active as thyroxine.

Substitution of bromine for iodine, namely, tetrabromothyronine,

$$HO \overline{\underset{Br}{\overset{Br}{\bigcirc}}} - O - \overline{\underset{Br}{\overset{Br}{\bigcirc}}} CH_2CHNH_2COOH,$$

gave a compound 3.0 percent, and a tetrachloro variety 0.2 percent, as active as thyroxine.

Thus it appears that the diphenyl structure is more important than having the right halogens, but also the right halogen is very important. Diiodothyronine is less active than tetrabromothyronine, but more so than tetrachlorothyronine.

Thyroxamine, a substance with the formula

$$HO \overset{I}{\underset{I}{\bigcirc}} -O- \overset{I}{\underset{I}{\bigcirc}} CH_2CH_2(NH_2),$$

tested by Gaddum,[19] has little or no activity, which would indicate that the carboxyl group is indispensable.

Alterations in the side chain, however, other than removing the carboxyl, seem of relatively less importance. Thus N-acetyl *l*-thyroxine,

$$HO \overset{I}{\underset{I}{\bigcirc}} -O- \overset{I}{\underset{I}{\bigcirc}} CH_2CHCOOH \\ NH_2COCH_3,$$

has 20 percent, and N-acetyl-d 1 thyroxyl-1-glutamic acid,

$$HO \overset{I}{\underset{I}{\bigcirc}} -O- \overset{I}{\underset{I}{\bigcirc}} CH_2CHNHCOCH_3 \\ CONHCHCH_2CH_2COOH, \\ COOH$$

has 5.5 percent the activity of *l*-thyroxine.

Methyl ether of thyroxine,

$$CH_3O \overset{I}{\underset{I}{\bigcirc}} -O- \overset{I}{\underset{I}{\bigcirc}} CH_2CHNH_2COOH,$$

also has about the same.

Of still less importance is the coupling of the carbon rings by a sulfur, instead of the usual oxygen, atom:

HO⟨ ⟩—S—⟨ ⟩$CH_2CHNH_2COOH.$ (each ring bearing two I atoms, top and bottom)

This gave a compound with 10.0 percent of the activity of *l*-thyroxine.

Thus it appears that nature has discovered that in order for the thyroid gland to accomplish its function with the greatest efficiency, a diphenyl alanine is essential, and, furthermore, that this must bear two or more atoms of a halogen, preferably iodine. The substitution of sulfur for oxygen in the coupling of the rings causes relatively slight deterioration in physiologic activity, and the same is true of certain alterations in the side chain.

Every component of the molecule seems to have its function, but just how this function is served remains obscure.

And now we come to the target. What influence does the hormone have upon the target, and how does it exert this influence?

We know in general terms that the target cell is speeded up in various ways. Its oxygen consumption is increased, and we also know that this increased consumption of oxygen is useful to the organism, that the energy released by the step oxidation of glucose is stored in high-energy phosphate compounds, and becomes available to the cell and the organism as needed. It is not all degraded into heat, and blown off, to the detriment of the cells or the organism, as is the case when a substance like dinitrophenol is administered.

It is unknown in what form thyroid hormone gains entry to the cell, whether as a free dissolved substance, or in some sort of peptide combination. Does it enter by simple diffusion? Probably it does, because Lipmann has found it in approximately the same concentration in intra- and extracellular fluid. There is no accumulation of it, as there is of iodine in the thyroid cell. Does it alter the permeability of the cell membrane with respect to other substances? What does it do after gaining entry to the cell, and what happens to the hormone in the process? At least it can be said that the hormone appears to be metabolized in the body, presumably in the same fashion as any amino acid. Certainly, too, it can be said that in some way it activates one or more of the enzyme systems of the cell. Lipmann has studied the distribution of thyroxine within the cell. Inasmuch as the mitochondria are known to be associated with the synthesis of adenosine triphosphate, it was anticipated that a higher concentration of thyroxine might be found within them, but such was not the case. Lipmann found it in about equal concentration in the nuclear fraction of his homogenates, the mitochondrial fraction, and the supernatant, which last represents the microsomes and soluble proteins of the cell.

One last point concerning the thyroid hormone which I should like to touch upon is the fundamental one of whether the output of hormone by the thyroid is determined by the call for hormone by the tissues, or whether the thyroid drives the tissues.

There are some bits of evidence which bear on this point. Rand, Riggs, and Talbot[20] exposed rats to cold long enough to cause stimulation of the thyroid. Then they determined the protein-bound iodine of the serum and compared it with that of rats which had been kept at room temperature. There was no difference. Dempsey and Astwood [21] have shown that when animals are exposed to cold more thyroid feeding is required to prevent thyroid enlargement than at room temperature. It appears, therefore, that under exposure to cold more thyroid hormone is put out, but that it does not pile up in the serum. From this it may be concluded that consumption of hormone is increased as much as production, which favors the theory that tissue cells are calling for hormone. If the thyroid gland were driving the cells, one would expect the protein-bound iodine of the serum to rise. All this is reminiscent of Barcroft's old concept of the call for oxygen by the tissues.

Harington in his Pedler Lecture (1944)[2] states that the terms of the lectureship require that "the lecture should indicate directions in which further work is required." I do not know that any such condition has been imposed in the case of the Thayer Lectures, but for this particular one, at least, it is not inappropriate. I will, therefore, close this discussion with certain suggestions as to how some of the gaps in our fragmentary knowledge of thyroid physiology might be narrowed. Actually I will mention five approaches, selected, be it understood, without any thought of ultimate practical value or application.

First, it seems to me that much more study of the iodide-trapping mechanism is indicated, and that this should be not alone from the point of view of the function of the thyroid gland, but with reference to, and for comparison with, other ion-trapping mechanisms of the body. It seems likely that the principle involved in iodide trapping by the thyroid is not fundamentally unique to the cells of that organ, but has its analogues in the functions of other tissues. The inquiry has now got to the stage, however, in which the physical chemist must come to the aid of the biological or medical investigator.

Second, it is important to discover the mechanism whereby the pituitary-thyroid axis is controlled, as it must be, from the higher levels of the nervous system. What is the neuro-humoral pathway involved?

Third, the metabolic cycle of thyrotropin should be worked out. How is this hormone produced, and what determines the response of its end-organs to it? We already know something of its excretion in both active and inactive form, but to get further on with the problem we badly need a method for determining its titer in the blood stream, and in other tissues, as easy of performance as is the eosinopenic response as applied to the quantitation of adrenocorticotropic activity.

My fourth suggestion is that an all-out effort be made to learn how thyroid hormone enters and affects its targets, and what happens to the hormone in the process. Is it consumed? Existing information indicates that it is, but how? It is not enough just to draw arrows from gland to target and let it go at that. Explorations in this area may well penetrate deeply into the fundamental nature of the act of living by the cell. It will require the services of enzymologists and physical chemists to solve this one.

Then also in the over-all end-organ problem is the fact that whereas thyroxine is a general somato-accelerator, when it comes to the cells of the anterior pituitary which are involved in thyrotropin production, it is an inhibitor, at least with respect to thyrotropic function. It also seems to be a direct inhibitor of the cells that make it, the thyroid parenchyma. These facts too need study. Nothing is known of the mechanism involved at present.

Lastly, I would dearly like to see explorations of the largely unplowed field of the phylogeny both of the thyroid gland and of its hormone. I expect that it will be found that the hormone antedated the gland. To the practically minded this approach may appear nebulous, but I cannot but believe that it may prove to be productive of new biological concepts. Below the verte-brates no recognizable thyroid tissue has been described, but there is some evidence, not very satisfactory, that vertebrate thy-roid may affect certain invertebrate species, even down to the level of the unicellular organisms. A search for all the iodine-bearing amino acids from protozoon to vertebrate might shed light on the evolution of thyroxine. It seems to me nature can only have perfected this efficient hormone, this streamlined mole-cule, after many trials with simpler structures. It is thus, I be-lieve, that the form of the living body and its component parts has come into being. Shall we not suppose that its biochemical anatomy has been similarly evolved? If it is worth while to trace the ancestry of an organ, why not that of a hormone also? The two combined will tell us the story of the organism.

3 The use of hormones, drugs, and radiations in the management of thyroid diseases

In this lecture let us shift our sights to a clinical level. Having now at our disposal a number of agents, the actions of which upon the thyroid gland are known, or partly known, in precise biological or biochemical terms, let us examine the various ways in which they can be applied in the care of patients with diseases of the thyroid gland or disturbances of thyroid function. These ways will include diagnosis as well as treatment. Instead of the usual clinical approach, namely, "How treat a given disease?" I wish to employ that of "Here is a tool; what is it good for?"

The tools I have grouped under the headings hormones, drugs, and radiations. I should perhaps have included surgical thyroid-ectomies, but that would have made the title too cumbersome. The diagnostic uses to which these tools can be put fall within the area of tests of function. The therapeutic uses fall within a certain framework which may be outlined as follows:

1. To suppress, or restrain, the pathologically overactive thyroid gland;
2. To augment the function of the pathologically underactive thyroid gland, or provide a substitute for it;
3. To alter the function of the normally acting thyroid in order to compensate for disturbed function elsewhere in the body (e.g., thyroidectomy or irradiation of the thyroid in certain cases of heart disease);
4. To remove or destroy mischievous thyroid tissue;

5. To obtain benefit through some extrathyroidal action of the agents in question (e.g., giving thyroid in the treatment of hyperophthalmopathic Graves's disease).

Let us keep this outline in mind as we proceed.

HORMONES

The hormones which I shall consider are thyroid hormone, thyrotropin, adrenocorticotropin, and adrenocortical hormone.

In the use of any of them I should like to distinguish sharply between physiological substitution therapy and pharmacotherapy. The former may be defined as the giving of a hormone, in cases of underactivity of an endocrine gland, in amount approximating what that gland would have made for itself under conditions of health. The pharmacotherapeutic use of hormones I should define as the giving of unphysiologically large doses of hormones, in order to obtain an alterative action which it is hoped may be beneficial to the patient. The administration of thyroid in myxedema is an example of the former; that of large doses of ACTH or cortisone in rheumatoid arthritis, lupus, pemphigus, or what have you, is an example of the latter. Physiologic substitution therapy, simply because it is physiologic, is without danger of untoward side effects. Pharmacotherapy with hormones is beset with much danger. In these days of fantastic, and sometimes even reckless, empiricism in hormone therapy, it is desirable that we pause occasionally to get our bearings.

Thyroid Hormone. Since the first successful use of any hormone was with thyroid, we may appropriately begin our discussion with that. Back in the early nineties it was discovered that the feeding of thyroid is a full, perfect, and sufficient therapy for the relief of myxedema (primary athyreosis) or Gull's disease. Parenteral exhibition of pure thyroxine is equally effective, but possesses no advantage over the oral administration of whole thyroid. All this, of course, is very ancient history, and I shall not belabor it further, except to stress one point, namely, that the relief of athyreosis by thyroid hormone is far more than merely raising the rate of energy metabolism. Dinitrophenol and related compounds have a profound calorigenic action, but Dodds and Robertson[1] have shown that the basal metabolic rate of a myxedematous subject can be raised from −20 to +70 by such a drug without there being any change whatever in the picture of athyreosis other than the rate of gas exchange. The action of thyroid hormone in physiologic dosage is utterly specific. No substances other than close chemical analogues of thyroxine can replace it, and analogues, except for triiodothyronine, must be given in far larger dosage than pure thyroxine to obtain a given effect.

There are uses, however, other than that of simple substitution therapy to which thyroid hormone can be put, and of these I wish now to speak. Instead, for example, of using it for its general somato-stimulatory action, it can be used for its inhibitory action on such targets as the pituitary and the thyroid gland itself. When in Graves's disease the ophthalmopathy takes on a malignant type of course, it is customary nowadays to give thyroid to tolerance, the rationale being that the lesion results from excessive thyrotropic activity on the part of the pituitary, and that thyroid hormone inhibits the pituitary with respect to its thyrotropic function. This is all very fine provided the premises are correct. I am confident that there is adequate evidence that thyroid hormone inhibits the pituitary with respect to thyrotropic activity, but the relation of thyrotropin to malignant exophthalmos is, to say the least, uncertain. There is, of course, the production of exophthalmos in animals by thyrotropin, and there is a little evidence indicating a high titer of thyrotropin in the blood in malignant exophthalmos. I have long suspected that changes in end-organ sensitivity, thyroid or orbital tissues, to thyrotropin, may play a role, but have no proof thereof. A great many patients with hyperophthalmopathic Graves's disease have been treated with thyroid, but so difficult is it to provide adequate control for clinical observations of this character that I am at a loss to say whether or not any benefit is conferred by such therapy. At least I am convinced that I have never seen any harm result from it, and that is more than can be said of many forms of therapy. I even have seen improvement occur, but whether the result of the therapy, or a spontaneous happening, I cannot say with any certainty. A statement made to me by Purves of New Zealand when he visited us in 1949 is very pertinent in this connection. He is one of the few who have made determinations of blood-thyrotropin level. He finds it elevated beyond normal in two conditions, myxedema and malignant exophthalmos. On the exhibition of thyroid in myxedema, blood-thyrotropin level promptly falls to normal; in malignant exophthalmos, however, even very large doses of thyroid fail to alter it. This finding could be interpreted to indicate that there is no sense in using thyroid in exophthalmos as it appears not to exert the action desired of it. Certainly a better pituitary inhibitor is needed. A few observations have been made on ACTH in this connection, but the results are equivocal.

Halsted years ago at Johns Hopkins showed that removal of a large part of a dog's thyroid is followed by hyperplasia of the fragment left in situ. This, we would now infer, must be due to increased thyrotropic activity of the pituitary. The giving of thyroid, or even of iodide, will prevent the development of hyperplasia of the thyroid remnant. Rienhoff,[2] also at Johns Hopkins, has made use of this principle to prevent the regrowth of toxic goiters after subtotal thyroidectomy. More recently Cope in our clinic has made use of thyroid therapy in a related manner. Observing that in hyperfunctioning adenomata of the thyroid the extranodular thyroid tissue tends to atrophy, he exhibited thyroid in cases of nontoxic goiter in order to bring any nodules that might be present into sharper relief by the expedient of causing atrophy of the extranodular thyroid tissue, so that the nature of the entire gland under study could be determined more accurately.

The use of thyroid in patients with habitually low basal metabolic rates, but lacking other evidence of hypothyroidism, needs mention. The etiology in such cases is really unknown, and the use of thyroid must be regarded as pharmacodynamic and empiric. Often the metabolic rate in such cases is relatively unaffected by thyroid. Occasionally one hears stories of such patients taking up to a gram of thyroid per day without its having much observable effect upon them. One interesting fact has been unearthed by Farquharson[3] as a result of such therapy. He found that after the metabolic rate in these patients has been elevated by means of heavy dosage of thyroid, if the hormone therapy is then suddenly terminated, the basal metabolic rate falls to a lower level than that from which it started before thyroid therapy. We have called this the Farquharson effect, and believe it due to thyroid hypoplasia resulting from an excess of extrinsic thyroid hormone. The administered thyroid could cause such an effect either by pituitary inhibition or by direct inhibition of the thyroid, or by a combination of these.

We have run into this area in another way — a way which involves the diagnostic use of basal metabolic rate, protein-bound iodine, and uptake of radioactive iodine. In spontaneous hyperthyroidism the values obtained by all these determinations are elevated. In true hypothyroidism they are all depressed. In thyrotoxicosis factitia, that is to say, due to ingestion of thyroid, basal metabolic rate and protein-bound iodine are elevated, but radioactive-iodine uptake is decreased, because the thyroid taken artificially causes hypoplasia or at least hypoactivity of the subject's own thyroid. Such a formula is of high diagnostic significance, and useful in the detection of patients who surreptitiously take thyroid.

As a diagnostic tool the exhibition of thyroid is of limited importance. If one had been unable to arrive at a positive diagnosis in a myxedemalike picture, the presence or absence of characteristic response to thyroid would be of diagnostic significance.

If, while being treated for definite hypothyroidism with thyroid, the patient went into Addisonian crisis, the diagnosis of hypothyroidism due to primary hypopituitarism would be established.

Thyroid, like the glamour hormones of today, has been tried in many diseases. Good results from such trials have been few and far between. There is, however, one that is rather striking, namely, the relief of certain cases of sterility and of habitual abortion in women by thyroid therapy.

So far as I am aware, the mechanism of the relief of sterility by thyroid is obscure. One is tempted to think that it may be a matter of acceleration of the energy transformation of the germ cells. On the relief of habitual abortion there is some evidence; Heinemann, Johnson, and Man,[4] for example, find that serum-precipitable iodine rises during pregnancy, and that this rise antedates the customary rise in basal metabolic rate. In women whose serum-precipitable iodine did not make the expected rise, abortion was likely. When such women received thyroid during pregnancy their SPI curve followed a normal course.

Goldsmith, Sturgis, Stanbury, and Lerman,[5] have made endometrial biopsies on women with untreated myxedema. Some of these had excessive bleeding and a few had no bleeding at all. Those with excessive menstrual flow were found to be bleeding from a proliferative, or estrogen-stimulated, endometrium. The others had atrophic endometria. In other words, these patients were not ovulating. In the cases of two men with untreated myxedema, testicular biopsies showed striking absence of Leydig cells. These findings suggest that in the myxedematous state the leutinizing hormone is not formed, and if the deficiency of thyroid is of sufficiently long standing, there may also be a failure of formation of the follicle-stimulating hormone by the anterior pituitary.

Thyrotropin. Although thyrotropin has been known longer than adrenocorticotropin, more is now known about the latter than about the former. The reason for this is probably twofold.

First, there is the widespread and intense interest in it which has resulted from the newly discovered and amazing pharmacodynamic action of cortisone, secretion of which hormone is promoted by ACTH. Second, there are easy quantitative tests for adrenocorticotropic action, such as the eosinopenic response, which are not available in the case of thyrotropic activity. Because of these circumstances it will be useful to bear the pituitary-cortical axis in mind as we consider the pituitary-thyroid.

When one wishes to bring about a remission in rheumatoid arthritis, he has a choice of two hormones, ACTH or cortisone. The effects of these on the patient as a whole are similar. In either case they are the result of increased supply of cortisone to the tissues. In one case the cortisone is given directly; in the other the patient's adrenal cortices are stimulated to put it out in increased quantity. It is a question of extrinsic supply of cortisone versus intrinsic. Although the effect on the patient's joint lesions may be identical in the two cases, that on his adrenal cortices is diametrically opposite. With ACTH his cortices are intensely stimulated; with cortisone they are put at rest.

Similar relations occur between thyroid hormone and thyrotropin. I have discussed the use of thyroid, and now the question becomes: do we ever need to use thyrotropin therapeutically or in diagnosis?

In primary myxedema substitution therapy with thyroid is as near perfection as any therapy I know. There would be no point in using thyrotropin in this condition because the atrophic thyroid probably could not respond to it. In a case of pananterior hypopituitarism, however, one might expect to restore thyroid function by means of thyrotropin, and secure as good a total effect as with thyroid. But there is no reason to suppose it would be better. In panhypopituitarism there is also hypofunction of the peripheral targets of other tropic hormones. The patient fundamentally needs a new anterior lobe. In the absence of this one can provide substitution therapy either by giving peripheral hormones, thyroid, cortisone, estrogens, etc., or by giving tropic hormones, thyrotropin, adrenocorticotropin, gonadotropins, etc. Whether one course is better than the other in biological terms I do not believe we know today. However the pituitary hormones presently available have the disadvantage that they may provoke antibody production. Moreover, for more than experimental use, thyrotropin is at present unavailable.

The only diagnostic use of thyrotropin that I can at present visualize is in cases in which it is desirable to know whether or not the patient's thyroid gland is capable of being stimulated. Such use would constitute one method of distinguishing between primary thyroidal myxedema and myxedema of pituitary origin. There are other methods of accomplishing this purpose. Querido and Stanbury[6] have made observations of this character in our clinic. They employed basal metabolic rate, protein-bound iodine, and radioactive-iodine uptake as criteria of thyrotropic effect. In five out of six cases of primary myxedema there was no evidence of response to thyrotropin as judged by any of these criteria. In a sixth there was an increase in protein-bound iodine and radioactive-iodine uptake following thyrotropin, but none in basal metabolic rate. In two cases judged to be of hypopituitarism on other grounds, there was marked increase in radioactive-iodine uptake and in protein-bound iodine after thyrotropin and in one a significant rise in basal metabolic rate also. Similar findings have been obtained by Perloff, Levy, and Despopoulas.[8]

The hypothesis has been raised that the so-called nonmyxedematous hypometabolic rate cases represent a condition of endorgan insensitivity, that is, insensitivity of their thyroid glands to the action of thyrotropin. Querido and Stanbury had one such case in their series. This patient made a good response to thyrotropin, which would be evidence against end-organ insensitivity, but of course much more is needed before any conclusion can be drawn.

Adrenocorticotropin (ACTH) and Cortisone. There is accumulating evidence that these hormones exert some depressant action on the activity of the pituitary-thyroid axis. Whether this is exerted at the pituitary level or at the thyroid level is not entirely clear, but the evidence favors the latter site of action. Depression of thyroid function in man following the administration of both ACTH and cortisone has been observed by several groups of workers. We observed six patients believed to have no thyroid disease during periods when they were receiving ACTH for other diseases. Four of these showed significant depression of I^{131} uptake and PBI, but none of the six showed any change in basal metabolic rate. The formula of decrease in I^{131} uptake and protein-bound iodine, but no change in basal metabolic rate, is an interesting one. A possible explanation would be that ACTH causes an increased sensitivity of somatic targets to thyroid hormone. Another is that these agents increased the renal clearance of iodide. Still another is that the glycocorticoids of themselves raise the BMR, which otherwise would be depressed. But there may be other explanations, although they do not occur to me at the moment. Another unexpected observation has been the usual, but not regular, failure of cortisone and ACTH to lower the indices of thyroid function in patients with Graves's disease. What does this imply concerning the pathological physiology of the clinical entity? I do not know.[7]

The use of cortical hormones in the toxic crises of Graves's disease (thyroid storm) antedates the introduction of cortisone. The nature of storm is still obscure, and as the condition is hardly ever met with in humans nowadays, and cannot be produced in animals, the chance of solving the problem is not bright. We still hold to the hypothesis that storm represents what may be called decompensated thyrotoxicosis. It seems likely that the adrenal cortex is hyperactive in hyperthyroidism and somewhat better evidence exists that it is hypoactive in hypothyroidism. The thyroid and the cortex seem to rise and fall together with respect to their functional activity. We have seen no literature on the eosinophile counts in storm, nor of autopsy material on the cortex either. Hyperthyroidism imposes a stress. The body responds to all stresses with adrenocortical hyperfunction. It could be that in thyroid storm the cortex becomes exhausted, and if this were true, it would be reasonable to administer cortical extract or cortisone.

DRUGS

The drugs I wish to consider are, on the one hand, iodine, and on the other, the growing group of so-called antithyroid or thyroinhibitor drugs. There are, of course, other drugs that are sometimes useful in the treatment of patients with diseases involving the thyroid gland—digitalis, quinidine, iron, vitamins, etc. — but the use of them is really not germane to the present discussion.

Iodine. It might be argued that iodine is not a drug at all, but a food, as are also iron and the other essential minerals. Certainly in the vertebrates from fish up, as shown by Marine, who started his career at Johns Hopkins, a minimal intake of iodine is essential to the preservation of health. The organism, whether fish or man, becomes goiterous when its iodine intake falls below a certain minimum, just as it becomes anemic with an inadequacy of iron, or asthenic during deprivation of salt, or osteomalacic when starved of calcium. The prophylaxis of goiter in regions where environmental iodine is scarce, by feeding iodine, could be said to fall within the field of dietetics rather than of pharmacology. It is only in high mountainous areas or postglacial regions of the earth that an external iodine shortage exists. In other parts there is invariably a superfluity of iodine so far as the needs of a normal organism are concerned; at least this is true unless there are present in the environment, simultaneously, positive goiter-producing factors.

It was undoubtedly Chesney and his collaborators (1928)[8] at Johns Hopkins who first clearly identified food factors as productive of goiter. Certain lots of cabbage were found to be the cause of an epidemic of goiter in his rabbit colony. Four years later Marine and his coworkers[9] showed that the food goitrogens were of the nature of cyanides, and all this recalled that back in 1905 Reid Hunt[10] had discovered the same phenomena in reverse, namely, that feeding thyroid protected animals against the toxic action of methylcyanide.

Twenty-three years elapsed between Hunt's discovery and Chesney's, and then it was another fourteen years before the great group of antithyroid drugs were added to our therapeutic equipment. Man learns slowly, but fortunately occasionally he learns. He might have argued in 1905, if thyroid protects against cyanide, perhaps cyanide will protect against thyroid, but he didn't.

I will not pursue further the dietetic use of iodine. Let us rather seek to identify its uses in the treatment of established disease.

First, there is the matter of established endemic goiter. If this is etiologically a pure iodine-want affair, will giving iodine cause it to regress? As is well known, usually it will not. Why? I believe the reason is something like this. Under long-continued iodine starvation, the thyroid, driven by the pituitary, becomes hyperplastic, and continues to make an abundance of thyroid protein, of thyroglobulin, even though it is unable to iodinate it. This iodine-poor colloid, being useless as hormone, is stored away in the follicles, which in consequence get ever larger and larger. The familiar colloid goiter is produced. Structural changes, cystic degeneration, involution, etc., occur in the gland which ultimately become irreversible. Even when adequate iodine is finally supplied the swollen gland is incapable of shrinking to its normal size. What may happen under such circumstances if iodine is given, is that the iodine-poor colloid is rapidly iodinated, and thyroxine is produced and discharged to the body in excess. The patient becomes temporarily thyrotoxic. This is what Kocher long ago called "Iod-Basedow." It is rarely if ever seen in the United States, but only in the highly goiterous areas of the world. (For further discussion of Iod-Basedow, see Lecture 5, pp. 96 and 97.)

The sporadic colloid goiters which one may encounter in non-endemic areas, and which differ anatomically from the endemic variety in no discernible way, may be due, as in the case of Stan-bury and Hedge's cretins, mentioned in the preceding lecture, to some intrinsic functional defect — inability to iodinate tyrosine or to couple diiodotyrosine to form thyroxine, or perhaps in certain cases to collect iodine at all. Giving iodine to such persons will have no beneficial effect. It will not overcome the block to hormone synthesis. Only the administration of thyroid can be expected to accomplish any useful purpose. When the gland cannot make hormone it must be given from without.

However, in certain cases of goiter due to ingestion of a goitrogenic agent, either as food, such as cabbage, or in the form of medicine, the exhibition of iodine may be curative.

For a time there was a vogue of treating hypertensives with thiocyanate. It is, I am sure, on the way out, as is sympathectomy, and probably soon the rice diet. This is just a prediction. The point is that patients treated with thiocyanate sometimes grew goiters, and when they did, the goiters could be made to go away, and also the hypothyroidism which accompanied them, by merely administering iodide. Thiocyanate seems to compete with iodide in the iodide-trapping mechanism, and an excess of iodide will prevent the uptake of thiocyanate, just as an excess of thiocyanate will prevent the uptake of iodide. Of course a still simpler program would be to stop giving the patient thiocyanate. If, on the other hand, a goiter were due to a drug of the thiouracil type, then giving iodide would be ineffectual because the primary difficulty under such circumstances would be in the iodination of tyrosine, not of collecting iodide.

The most important therapeutic use of iodine in thyroid disease, aside from that in the prevention or correction of iodine-want goiter, is in Graves's disease. The well-known response to iodine of the thyrotoxicosis in that malady remains, so far as cause and mechanism go, pretty much a mystery. This response and its mechanism have interested me for many years, ever since 1923 in fact, when Plummer brought it to the attention of the profession. In 1938 Lerman and I[11] analyzed the curve described by the basal metabolic rate of patients with thyrotoxic Graves's disease during the administration of iodine. We compared it with the so-called thyroxine decay curve of Boothby and others, and found it to be altogether similar. From this we concluded that the action of iodine in Graves's disease is to stop, at least temporarily, the release of thyroid hormone from the thyroid gland. How this effect is exerted, or why it occurs in thyrotoxic patients but not in normal persons, remains entirely obscure. In 1945 several of us made the observation that even when the thyroids of patients with Graves's disease are blocked with thiouracil, they still undergo involution when iodine is administered. In other words, it appeared that the iodinating action of iodine had been divorced from an involuting action. Again the explanation is not clear, but some later work of Rawson's, done while he was with us, may illuminate it somewhat. Rawson found in the first place that when thyrotropin acts upon the thyroid, it becomes physiologically inactivated. Later he showed that iodine interferes with the inactivation of thyrotropin by slices of thyroid, and that it inhibits the action of thyrotropin in hypophysectomized rats. Finally he found that patients with untreated Graves's disease excreted no active thyrotropin in their urine, but that after treatment with iodine they did excrete some. It was as though the untreated hyperactive gland was inactivating thyrotropin energetically, but that iodine interfered with this process and active thyrotropin spilled out in the urine.

Going back now to the nature of the iodine response in Graves's disease in the light of Rawson's last-mentioned work, it may be that the divorce of iodinating and involuting action may be explained by the theory that iodine blocks the action of thy-rotropin in thyroid cells, thus stopping thyroxine manufacture, but the thyroid cells go on manufacturing protein which piles up in the follicles and is not withdrawn therefrom, having no hor-monic value. This theory does not explain why iodine does not have a similar action in normals, but concerning that another finding of Rawson's was that thyroids from patients with thyro-toxic Graves's disease inactivate more thyrotropin than normals. A change in end-organ sensitivity to thyrotropin may be at the bottom of the matter.

So specific to Graves's disease is the iodine response that in earlier days we used it as a diagnostic test. Now with the newer diagnostic measures available, this seldom is necessary.

In treatment of thyrotoxicosis nowadays we seldom use iodine alone, but we do use it in combination with an antithyroid drug, in the preparation of thyrotoxic patients for operation.

Antithyroid Drugs. As I have already indicated, these fall into at least two categories, those which block the iodine-trapping mechanism, and those which block the synthetic process. The former are the thiocyanate ions and perchlorate, and the latter thiourea and its analogues, and some other substances with sim-ilar action.

Diagnostically these drugs may be used, as in the case of the cretins cited previously, to determine the location of a defect in the assembly line of hormone biosynthesis.

When it comes to therapeutics it may be said that, thus far, sulfocyanate does not appear to be of great importance. It might, to be sure, be used in controlling thyrotoxicosis, as suggested by Chapman before the advent of the thioureas, but it is inferior to the latter for that purpose. However, perchlorate has been suc-cessfully used in controlling Graves's disease, thus far without untoward effects, and with an efficiency comparable to the thiou-rea derivatives.[12]

The thiourea analogues, of course, have made a great stir in the treatment of thyrotoxicosis, especially that of Graves's disease. They have also been used to produce hypothroidism as treatment for certain forms of cardiac insufficiency. A huge amount of pharmacologic work has been done on these drugs with a view to improvement in the molecule with respect to greater antithyroid action and at the same time lessened tendency to produce toxic side effects. It has been, one might say, a process of pharmacologic streamlining. It is not my intention here to discuss the relative merits of the several drugs that have been tried. I am at present only concerned with the question, what have these drugs in general to offer in the treatment of thyroid diseases? In actual thyroid diseases, besides for thyrotoxicosis, they have been tried, so far as I know, only in the treatment of thyroiditis, and it is my belief that for the latter purpose they really offer nothing. They also are used to produce hypothyroidism, when it is thought that hypothyroidism may be beneficial.

They are used widely as definitive therapy in Graves's disease, and to a lesser extent in toxic adenomatous goiter. For the latter they are certainly inferior to surgical thyroidectomy. As definitive treatment in Graves's disease I personally do not like them as well as either radioactive iodine or surgical thyroidectomy. To get permanent remission of thyrotoxicosis in Graves's disease one must usually continue the administration of these drugs without interruption for at least a year, and even then one often fails in one's objective. Surgical thyroidectomy removes thyroid tissue and radioactive iodine destroys it in situ, but the antithyroid drugs merely hold it in functional abeyance. To be sure, if such control is exerted long enough, the disease may go into spontaneous remission during the period of treatment.

RADIATIONS

Radiations are used in cases of thyroid disease, both in diagnosis and in treatment. In treatment they are used, both x-ray and radioactive isotopes, for the purpose of destroying thyroid tissue either hyperplastic or neoplastic. Radium itself has been so used, but very infrequently, and hardly at all at present, so I will not say more about it. X-ray in treatment is hardly ever used nowadays in thyrotoxicosis, and in cancer it is only used in those cases in which all the malignant tissue cannot be removed and will not take up iodine.

In diagnosis x-ray is used to delineate goiters and demonstrate metastases. This use is familiar enough, and needs no further comment. Radioactive isotopes, chiefly of iodine, are used as tracers to see where they go and the extent of their uptake. In addition to iodine, other isotopes may be used as tracers. Rawson has labeled thyrotropin with sulfur.

Radioactive Iodine. Radioactive iodine, chiefly I^{131}, has been extensively used in experimental work, notably by Hertz, Rawson, Chaikoff, LeBlond, Keating, Skanse, Dobyns, Stanbury, and others. I have touched upon some of this in the preceding lecture. I will not go further with it at present; instead let us consider the diagnostic situation.

Briefly the tracer situation can be said to resolve itself as follows: (1) the determination by direct scanning of uptake by the thyroid gland itself or by distant thyroid tissue; (2) excretion — calculation of thyroid uptake by difference; (3) concentration and partition in the blood; (4) cytologic localization of iodine in the thyroid gland, or autoradiography.

The determination of total uptake of radioiodine by the thyroid is useful diagnostically, chiefly in ruling hyper- or hypothyroidism in or out. It is highly instructive to compare it with simultaneous determinations of the level of protein-bound iodine in the blood and basal metabolic rate. In spontaneous thyrotoxicosis all three values are elevated. In thyrotoxicosis factitia the basal metabolic rate and protein-bound iodine are elevated. Uptake of radioactive iodine is depressed. The reasons for this were discussed in the preceding lecture. In phaeochromocytoma the basal metabolic rate may be elevated, but protein-bound iodine and radioactive iodine uptake would not be. The explanation here is that the hypermetabolism is due to adrenalin, not to thyroxine.

In vivo, localized regional scanning is particularly valuable in determining the functional activity of thyroid nodules as compared with the remaining extranodular and thyroid tissue. Some nodules can be shown to collect more radioactivity than intranodular tissue, some less. In some cases there is little difference between them. We have dropped into the habit of calling those nodules which take up iodine briskly, "hot nodules"; those which do not we call "cold nodules." There are, to be sure, a certain number of lukewarm nodules. Information of this character is diagnostically useful because there is a relatively high percentage of cancer in single nodules (18 percent of all single nodules in our series). Single nodules are the easiest to scan directionally. Cancers take up less iodine than extranodular tissue. If a hot nodule is found, one can assume that the chance of its being malignant is negligible. On the other hand, the finding that a nodule is cold raises an impressive possibility of malignancy. With such knowledge in advance the surgeon is better prepared to deal with malignancy if he finds it. He starts his operation ready to do a radical resection if indicated.

In older patients with heart disease the finding of a hot nodule suggests a hyperthyroid etiology, and raises the possibility of very marked relief by thyroidectomy.

Autoradiography locates function and correlates it with structure. We are getting new concepts of the significance of cytologic pictures. For example, certain hyperplastic adenomas are functionless while others with minimal hyperplasia may function actively. Many tumors which are forming colloid are not necessarily turning over iodine. Just because colloid is seen does not mean that the tumor can take up iodine. In this connection one is reminded of the divorce of iodinating action of iodine and its involuting action in Graves's disease which I mentioned earlier.

Treatment of Graves's disease by means of radioactive iodine

has been under study in our clinic for ten years. In Hertz's original series there were 29 cases. Naturally in the beginning con-
servative dosage of radiation was employed with the result that
in some of the cases control of thyrotoxicosis was incomplete and
surgical thyroidectomy was performed later. Since 1943 Earle M.
Chapman has had the assignment, and under his observations 315
patients with Graves's disease and 10 with toxic nodular goiter
have been treated. Of these only four have subsequently required
surgery. Fifteen have been overtreated and required thyroid therapy. In three of them hypothyroidism was purposely produced
because of accompanying heart disease.

Of the four patients that were operated on, the case of one was
particularly instructive. This patient had Graves's disease, but
with two incidental nodules. One of these was biopsied and found
to be benign. Therefore the patient was treated with radioactive
iodine, which relieved her thyrotoxicosis. However, the remaining
nodule, left in situ, persisted and caused some worry. It was
accordingly removed and turned out to be carcinomatous. There
was no way of knowing whether the irradiation had anything to
do with its becoming malignant. It is believed that the surgical
resection removed all the malignant tissue.

This case caused us to establish the policy of not treating nodular goiters with radioactive iodine.

Another worry was over the case of a patient from New Bruns-
wick. She was treated with radioactive iodine for Graves's disease
five years ago. Very recently we were informed that she had died
of malignant disease believed primary in her thyroid and with
multiple bone metastases. Some sections of both thyroid and
bone lesions were sent to us, and our pathologists were quite
certain that the case was one of multiple myeloma — not of thy-
rogenic cancer.

A third patient treated for Graves's disease with radioactive
iodine died of widespread bronchogenic cancer with one small
metastasis in the thyroid, but no patient in the whole series, so

far as we know, has developed primary cancer of the thyroid. The late biopsies which have been performed show fibrosis and regenerative hyperplasia. In some areas bizarre nuclear changes were seen but no unequivocal evidence or malignancy.

Still we are worried about the possibility of producing cancer, and only until more years elapse and more patients are treated shall we feel that this ghost has been laid permanently.

A somewhat encouraging therapeutic use of radioactive iodine is in the treatment of certain cancers of the thyroid. Of course in any type of thyroid cancer, as with any other cancer, the indication is to remove all malignant tissue surgically if that is possible. When it is not possible, radioactive iodine can be used if the tumor will take up, or can be induced to take up, iodine. When no iodine uptake can be developed, then x-ray therapy is all that remains. Destruction of malignant thyroid tissue by radioiodine is to be preferred to x-ray, being more selective.

One would like to think that the I^{131} effect can be pin-pointed on the target to a far greater extent than with x-ray. The destruction to tumor would therefore be maximal, and injury to other tissues minimal. At present we fall far short of our wishes, because there are wide variations in the concentration density of the isotope even within the same metastasis, leaving gaps of tumor tissue which cannot be bridged by the beta ray of the I^{131}.

The plan of attack developed by Cope and Dobyns of our clinic is as follows: A tracer dose of radioactive iodine is always given preoperatively. If cancer is encountered, its iodine-collecting capacity is determined by autoradiography of the excised tissue or by digestion of this and counting thereafter. If cancer tissue cannot be completely removed, then all normal thyroid tissue is removed. A gamma-ray counter can be used at the operation in the search for thyroid tissue. All tissue showing an uptake is removed. The reason for this tactic is to place the burden of thyroid-hormone production entirely on the remaining cancer. Such a maneuver may induce it to take up iodine. That is to say, a nonfunctioning cancer may be converted into a functioning one. If this can be accomplished, radioiodine therapy may be employed with some hope of success. An example of this is shown in Fig. 3.

Our best results have been obtained in cases of the follicular type of adenocarcinoma, particularly distant metastatic lesions. In only a minority of papillary carcinomas can an iodine uptake be developed. Undifferentiated cancers seldom develop an iodine uptake, or at least kill the patient before an uptake can be developed.

Since 1946 we have studied about 120 thyroid cancers with I^{131}. A handful of these with well-differentiated tumors have shown sufficient concentrating capacity for the isotope to give any promise of benefit. The most impressive effects are in the bone lesions, and one patient, Mrs. D., has shown complete clearing of multiple pulmonary metastases. The bone lesions may remain, but stop growing, and the patients may become asymptomatic.

I will mention three other cases very briefly and then have done.

Mrs. M., with follicular adenocarcinoma of the thyroid, had a metatastasis to the humerus, with a pathologic fracture, and another in her ilium with limitation of motion in her leg. After radioactive-iodine treatment the arm has healed, and she has regained good function of her leg.

Mr. B. had a total thyroidectomy for cancer in 1946. He had metastatic disease in his spine with collapsed vertebrae and much pain. He is asymptomatic today with his cancer held in abeyance by radioactive iodine and his spine splinted by a successful bone graft.

Mrs. S.'s presenting symptomatology was pain in her right hip and buttock which caused a significant impediment to walking. By x-ray a destructive lesion of the bony pelvis was found and by biopsy it proved to be of thyroid origin. A parent lesion was

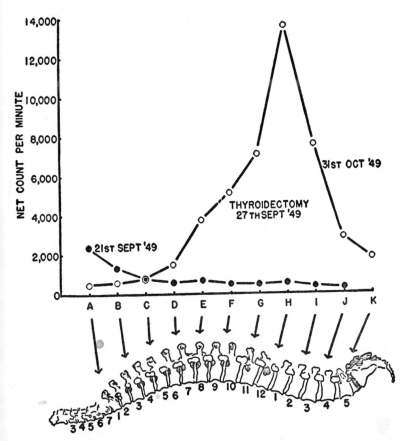

Fig. 3. Effect of thyroidectomy on the avidity for iodine of a metastatic thyroid cancer in the lower dorsal spine (D11 and D12). The diagram indicates uptake of I^{131} over the several spinal segments before total thyroidectomy (black dots) and 34 days afterward (circles). The ordinate shows the Geiger-counter readings. It will be observed that a considerable iodine uptake was developed over the lesion after thyroidectomy.

found in the thyroid gland. A total thyroidectomy was performed. Following this the metastasis developed an iodine uptake, and radioactive iodine therapy was used. As a result of this the bone lesion has been restrained and her symptoms have disappeared.

In conclusion I may say that what I have outlined are the chief measures we have today for controlling or modifying the activity of the thyroid gland within the body. Always it should be understood that such control is exercised exclusively for the good of the patient as a whole. Neither the thyroid nor any other organ is a therapeutic objective in itself. We may expect, as in any field, that if we engage in research, our methods of control will continuously be modified and improved.

4 Clues to the etiology of Graves's disease

Though hyperthyroidism is usually present at some stage of Graves's disease this is not to be regarded as a relatively simple endocrinopathy like primary athyreosis or Gull's disease; it is a widespread and complex constitutional disorder involving, besides the thyroid, other endocrine glands, the tissues of the orbit, the spleen, the thymus, and the lymphatic, reticuloendothelial, hemopoietic, muscular, nervous, and very likely other bodily systems.

The etiology of Graves's disease is a challenging subject for inquiry, and, particularly as regards its ocular manifestations, its treatment presents an urgent problem for the clinician. I cannot offer any solutions; I can merely make surmises and indicate approaches already being used and clues which it may be profitable to follow in the future.

In Gull's disease the primacy of the thyroid gland, if we may use that term in a negative sense, is indisputable. The gland has undergone atrophy or been destroyed, and all the manifestations of the disease may be interpreted as the result, direct or indirect, of lack of thyroid hormone throughout the body. One cannot with equal confidence assert that Graves's disease is essentially the opposite. The primacy of the thyroid gland in Graves's disease has never been conclusively established.

If we wish to see simple hyperthyroidism we can feed thyroid gland to normal people, or we can find it occurring naturally in cases of oversecreting thyroid adenoma. As a background to our inquiry into the nature of Graves's disease, it may be well to examine this seemingly simpler disturbance.

TOXIC ADENOMA OF THE THYROID

The late Henry S. Plummer,[1] of the Mayo Clinic, was chiefly responsible for distinguishing between toxic adenoma of the thyroid and Graves's disease, or exophthalmic goiter, as he preferred to call it, and for regarding them as of different origin. For many years I doubted the validity of this distinction. I never denied the existence of toxic adenoma; indeed, I admitted that, since there were plenty of instances of oversecreting tumors in other endocrine glands, it was reasonable to expect them in the thyroid. However, I failed to discover, in my clinic, cases which on clinical grounds I could confidently call Plummer's disease rather than Graves's disease. The thyrotoxic patients with nodules in their thyroid glands I took to be cases of Graves's disease with goiters which happened to be nodular.

The advent of radioactive iodine has entirely changed this interpretation. We have proved with this agent that true oversecreting tumors may occur in the thyroid, and that the hyperthyroidism they produce is etiologically distinct from that of Graves's disease. The tumor alone oversecretes in Plummer's disease, the whole gland in Graves's disease.

It is highly probable that the activities of all tissues, except true neoplasms, are under either nervous or humoral control, or both. Neoplasms are almost certainly not under nervous control, and it seems likely that they have also largely escaped from humoral control.

Investigation of Function. The function of thyroid adenomata can be studied by giving the patient tracer doses of radioactive iodine. It is well established now by extensive investigations on animals that the uptake of labeled iodine by the thyroid gland is a dependable index of the rate of secretory activity of the thyroid cells. Uptake after administration of tracer doses can be determined in at least three ways: scanning over the region of the thyroid with an externally applied gamma-ray detector is the most direct way; excision of thyroid tissue and the making of auto-radiograms with tissue slices is another; and a third, indirect, method is to determine what proportion of the administered dose of radioactivity is excreted in the urine, and then to assume that the remainder has been retained for the most part by the thyroid gland. Still another method is that of Seed, who determines the "conversion ratio," or the rate at which the gland can remove a tracer of radioactive iodide from the blood and return it to the blood in protein-bound form.

When one applies these methods to the study of thyroid tumors, the results range from that in which a tumor takes up no iodine, and hence is to be regarded as totally inactive, to one in which a tumor takes up iodine with great avidity and the remainder of the thyroid takes up little or none.

Malignancy. In the thyroid gland, as in most other tissues, both benign and malignant tumors may be found. Whether the malignant tumors only originate in the benign or may arise de novo from previously normal tissue is unknown. There is plenty of evidence that benign thyroid tumors may ultimately become malignant. But it is also apparent that malignant tumors usually secrete only slightly, if at all, whereas benign ones may secrete enough to produce hyperthyroidism, and when they have done so the possibility of their becoming also malignant is remote. Indeed, it is extremely rare to find cancer in the thyroid gland of any thyrotoxic persons, whether the source of their hyperthyroidism is a tumor or the diffuse hyperplasia of Graves's disease. For many years we considered hyperthyroidism a good guarantee against thyroid cancer. Recently we have found histologically malignant nodules buried in the hyperplastic thyroids in several cases of Graves's disease; none of them formed metastases, and what might have happened to them had they remained in situ cannot be said. In spite of this experience we still believe that,

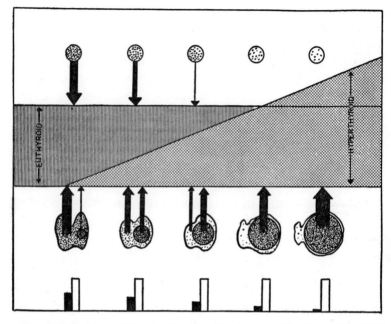

Fig. 4. Life history of secreting thyroid adenoma ("hot" nodule). The upper row of circles represents the anterior lobe of the pituitary gland; intensity of stippling and width of arrows indicate the degree of thyrotropic activity.

The lower row of circles, enlarging from left to right, denotes the growth of the tumor in the thyroid gland; intensity of stippling denotes functional activity disclosed by uptake of radioactive iodine. Arrows, by their thickness, indicate contribution of thyroid hormone by both the tumor and the remainder of the thyroid gland.

The single-hatched zone indicates the portion of the basal metabolic rate produced by hormone from nonneoplastic thyroid parenchyma, and the cross-hatched zone that by hormone from the tumor.

The columns at the base represent cell height: black, of thyroid parenchyma; white, of tumor.

to a large extent, hyperplasia and malignant neoplasia are mutually exclusive. The significance of this relation is not yet apparent, but it may later become so. It is worth bearing in mind.

Life History of Adenoma. The life history of the oversecreting thyroid nodule has been well worked out in our clinic with radioactive iodine. The important phases are shown diagrammatically in Fig. 4. Here is portrayed an adenoma which produces thyroid hormone from its birth onward. In the beginning it is very small and its contribution of hormone is insignificant compared with that of the rest of the gland. The thyroid gland, as the diagram shows, is under pituitary control, making just enough total hormone to maintain the patient in a euthyroid state. However, the tumor grows out of control and, as it does so, contributes more and more hormone in simple relation to the total volume of its parenchyma. The pituitary gland, we suspect (it has not been proved), in these circumstances restricts its output of thyroid-stimulating hormone so that as the tumor produces more and more hormone, the remainder of the thyroid, in compensation, makes less and less. Finally, as the tumor grows, the time comes when it alone makes enough thyroid hormone to keep the patient in a euthyroid state. At this point, we suspect, on the basis of what is actually known of pituitary-thyroid balance, that the pituitary gland ceases altogether to produce thyroid-stimulating hormone, and the normal thyroid parenchyma consequently becomes atrophic and functionless. However, the process does not stop here. The tumor, being out of control, continues to grow and make even greater quantities of thyroid hormone. The patient therefore at last becomes thyrotoxic and enters a stage in which he can be truly said to have a toxic adenoma of the thyroid.

This diagrammatic simplification (Fig. 4) is based not only on collections of radioiodine by the thyroid and basal metabolic rates but also on measurements of the mean acinar cell height of the thyroid parenchyma. The extensive studies of Rawson and Starr[2] have demonstrated a close relation between the height of thyroid cells and their functional activity. Dobyns and Lennon[3] have shown that the same holds true, usually but not always, for the epithelium of thyroid tumors. In Fig. 4 I have therefore indicated cell heights as well as function estimated from iodine collections. The height of the tumor cells, it will be seen, is above that of the

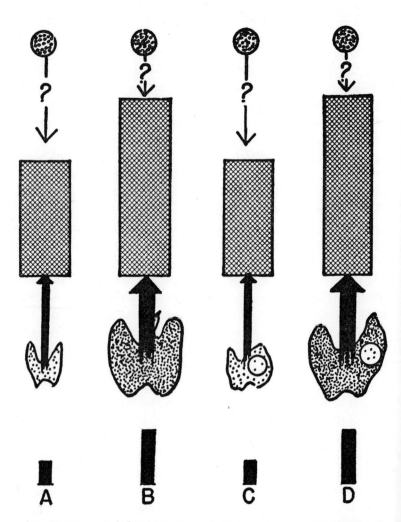

Fig. 5. Hormonic relations in Graves's disease as compared with normal, with or without incidental "cold" nodule, constructed in similar fashion to Fig. 4. The heights of the cross-hatched rectangles indicate basal metabolic rates; the columns at the base denote heights of thyroid acinar cells: *A*, normal thyroid; *B*, Graves's disease with thyrotoxicosis; *C*, normal thyroid with incidental nodule; *D*, Graves's disease with incidental nodule.

normal cells from the beginning and remains fixed at this high level, whereas that of the normal cells steadily declines as the tumor takes over and the pituitary gland restricts its output of thyrotropic hormone.

The situation in Graves's disease is altogether different. Here we have no evidence that the thyroid parenchyma escapes from hormonic control. Unless, perchance, the sensitivity of thyroid cells as end-organs is altered, which is possible but not proved, we may assume that the thyroid abnormality in Graves's disease lies in the control of the thyroid gland rather than in the gland itself.

Pituitary-thyroid Axis. Salter[4] referred to the pituitary-thyroid relation as the pituitary-thyroid axis, and this is a convenient term to use. The pituitary gland makes a hormone that stimulates the thyroid gland to make its hormone, which in turn inhibits the pituitary gland. It may be regarded as, within limits, an automatic physiologic mechanism. As I conceive the situation in toxic adenoma of the thyroid, it is one in which the axis functions ably to preserve the euthyroid state of the patient until the limit of its ability to effect an adjustment is reached. Only at this point does the patient become thyrotoxic. In the thyrotoxicosis of Graves's disease, on the other hand, I regard the axis as out of kilter from the beginning or as receiving a morbid signal from the hypothalamus.

In Fig. 5 I have indicated these relations. Here we have parallel increases in iodine uptake, thyroid size, cell height, and basal metabolic rate. All these may be due to increased thyrotropic activity of the pituitary gland, or possibly to increased sensitivity of the thyroid target to its pituitary stimulator. If the latter were the case one would expect compensation for a time until it reached its limit. Whether such compensation occurs needs determining. An approach seems to be to discover what really is the normal stimulus to the thyrotropic function of the pituitary gland. Is it the absolute level of thyroid hormone in the blood, the basal metabolic rate of the patient, or what? The answer to this question may provide a clue to the etiology of Graves's disease.

Results Obtained with Radioiodine. In Fig. 5 I have also indicated one of the reasons for my skepticism, before the days of radioiodine, about the existence of toxic thyroid adenoma. Graves's disease may occur in persons with nonsecreting nodules in their thyroids; this condition would be correctly called, descriptively, toxic nodular goiter, but it is really Graves's disease with incidental thyroid nodule or nodules, neoplastic or other. Before radioiodine came along, such situations made for confusion; now by its use we can very easily separate secreting from nonsecreting nodules and thus understand the morbid process more accurately. In our clinic we call secreting nodules "hot" and nonsecreting nodules "cold," and for convenience I shall use that terminology from here on.

The sort of thing one finds on scanning the neck with the directional gamma-ray detector after a tracer dose of radioiodine, in the several conditions I have been talking about, is shown in Fig. 6. The circles indicate the location of the aperture of the counter, and the numerals indicate the number of detected nuclear disintegrations per minute observed in those areas. When the normal value is 200–400 counts per minute, the value in Graves's disease may be 10–20 times as high. The number of counts partly depends on the thickness of thyroid tissue just beneath the counter. Therefore in interpreting results one must give some weight to anatomy.

The upper left-hand diagram shows what one might find over a normal thyroid gland, and the diagram next to it the sort of result found with the diffusely hyperplastic gland in Graves's disease. The third diagram shows the thyroid gland in Graves's disease with an incidental nodule. The nodule here, the masses of tissue involved being taken into consideration, does not take up a significantly greater amount of iodine than does the rest of the parenchyma. It is a relatively cold nodule, or certainly not more than a lukewarm one. The fourth and fifth diagrams show typical examples of hot and cold nodules in otherwise normal thyroids. The hot nodule, though located at an upper pole where counts tend normally to be low, gives a significantly higher value than

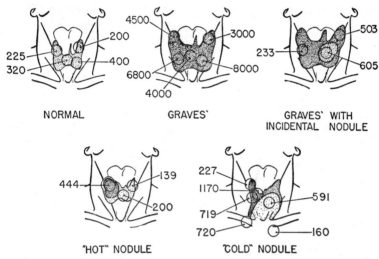

Fig. 6. Results of scanning of the neck with a directional gamma-ray counter after a tracer dose of radioiodine. The numbers indicate counts per minute recorded over the areas indicated. The aperture of the counter was 1.9 centimeters in diameter. The upper left-hand diagram indicates the findings from a normal thyroid gland. The next diagram is a result found with the diffusely hyperplastic gland of Graves's disease. The third shows the findings in Graves's disease with an incidental nodule. The fourth and fifth diagrams represent typical examples of "hot" and "cold" nodules in otherwise normal glands.

does the remaining parenchyma, whereas the cold nodule, though a large mass of tissue, gives a lower value than any area except the right upper pole, where a low value would be expected.

Dobyns, Skanse, and Maloof[5] have used the ratio of iodine collection by nodules to collection by extranodular thyroid tissue to distinguish between secreting and nonsecreting lesions. Any

value for this ratio above 2 they regard as denoting an oversecreting nodule.

Relation of Iodine Collection to Parenchymal Cell Height. This
is of interest both in nonneoplastic and in neoplastic tissue. As
I mentioned earlier, we had concluded, on the work of Rawson
and Starr,[2] that cell height is a good index of thyroid activity.
Increase in cell height denoted cellular hypertrophy, and hypertrophy was an accompaniment of oversecretion. This conclusion
is probably justified so far as nonneoplastic tissue is concerned,
but Dobyns, Skanse, and Maloof [5] have measured the heights of

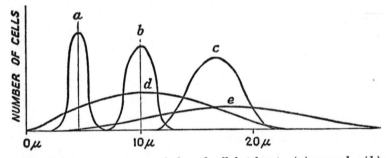

Fig. 7. Frequency curves of thyroid-cell heights in (*a*) normals, (*b*)
Graves's disease, (*c*) oversecreting adenoma ("hot" nodule), (*d*) under-
secreting adenoma ("cold" nodule), and (*e*) adenocarcinoma. (After
Dobyns.)

the epithelial cells of thyroid tumors and find some departures
from the rule governing nonneoplastic tissue. In brief, they find
in some tumors cells which are high but inactive. In an effort to
solve this riddle they studied not only mean cell height but also
distribution curves of cell height. The gist of their findings,
smoothed a bit, is shown in Fig. 7. Here we have frequency
curves of thyroid acinar cell height similar to those of Price Jones
on erythrocyte diameter: (*a*) in normal thyroids, (*b*) in Graves's
disease, (*c*) in an oversecreting thyroid adenoma (hot nodule),
(*d*) in an undersecreting or nonsecreting adenoma, and (*e*) in
an adenocarcinoma of the thyroid.

It appears from these curves that relative uniformity in cell height is characteristic of normal and of nonneoplastic hyperplastic tissue. Increasing variability in cell height marks the transition from normal or simple hyperplastic tissue to neoplastic tissue, and the cells of secreting neoplastic tissue vary less in height than those of nonsecreting neoplastic tissue.

GRAVES'S DISEASE

Ophthalmopathy. One of the most amazing manifestations of Graves's disease is the ophthalmopathy; what on earth can it have to do with the thyroid? There are syndromes due to oversecretion by other nonneoplastic endocrine glands — adrenal cortex, parathyroid, gonad, etc. — but none of these, so far as I know, includes anything as bizarre or apparently unrelated to the function of the primarily involved endocrine gland as is the ophthalmopathy of Graves's disease. I always react vigorously when the eye signs are enumerated among the signs of thyrotoxicosis. They are not signs of thyrotoxicosis, because they may progress when the patient is in a hypothyroid phase. I think the most reasonable position to take is that ophthalmopathy and thyrotoxicosis are both manifestations of Graves's disease, but that one is in no sense the result of the other. Either may be lacking at some stage of the disease in any given case.

Since exophthalmos was first produced by injections of anterior-pituitary extracts, it has generally been believed that an excessive production of thyrotropic hormone plays some important role in its pathogenesis. But, if this is true, how is it that ophthalmopathy and thyrotoxicosis in Graves's disease can vary independently, or at least in nonparallel fashion? This dilemma brings to mind the question of end-organ sensitivity, and perhaps also of chalones which might antagonize the action of thyrotropic hormone. The only proved end-organ of thyrotropic hormone, so far as I know, is the thyroid parenchyma. If the tissues of the orbit are also specific end-organs for this hormone, it seems a remarkable relation. The growth hormone, and perhaps the diabetogenic hormone and fat-mobilizing hormone, act on non-endocrine targets, but otherwise the tropic hormones of the pituitary gland act, seemingly, only on other endocrine glands.

The work of Rawson and Starr[2] on thyrotropic hormone indicates that its first action on the thyroid gland is to accelerate the release of thyroid hormone. In serving this function it becomes physiologically inactivated, but by treatment with mild reducing agents its activity can be restored. As regards the inactivation of thyrotropic hormone, Rawson and Starr also made two other discoveries which may be of deep significance: (1) the thyroid glands of patients with Graves's disease can inactivate more thyrotropic hormone than can those of normal people; and (2) besides the thyroid gland, lymph-node tissue and thymus gland can likewise inactivate thyrotropic hormone.

Warthin[6] attached great importance to the involvement of lymphoid tissue in Graves's disease. He claimed that it constituted the most striking feature of the histopathology of the disease, and he looked on it as an expression of a constitutional state of the thymicolymphatic type which he called the "Graves's constitution." Unless one were born with this, so Warthin claimed, one would never get exophthalmic goiter. I am not prepared to accept Warthin's contentions unreservedly, but I am to some degree in sympathy with them. There can be small doubt that inheritance plays some role in Graves's disease; also it is impressive that lymphoid high lights keep appearing, first in one place and then in another, in the over-all picture.

When Rawson and Starr found that lymph-node tissue, as well as thyroid and thymus tissue, would inactivate thyrotropic hormone, I at once thought of Warthin's old theory. I also recalled that in the ophthalmopathy of Graves's disease the ocular muscles are invaded by lymphocytes — indeed, actual lymphorrhages may be found in them. All these facts concerning lymphatic tissue in Graves's disease must be related and must have some significance, but what it may be I cannot tell. Perhaps, however, Warthin was right, and here may lie one clue, at least, to the enigma of Graves's disease. Certainly the lymphatic component deserves further and vigorous study, and so does the muscular component. It is well known that some patients present a myopathy not merely in the orbit but also throughout the entire skeletal muscular system. Instead of the orbits being selectively involved, it is possible that the state of affairs there is merely a local exaggeration of a widespread process, conditioned by local peculiarities.

In any event, in my own thinking, I keep returning to the orbit. I cannot escape a strong conviction that the solution to the problem it presents may solve that of the whole disease. The production of exophthalmos in animals with pituitary extracts seems a very important clue, but it is disconcerting (1) that none of the preparations of thyrotropic hormone thus far used are completely pure, which fact leaves open the possibility of their containing an exophthalmos-producing substance other than thyrotropic hormone; and (2) that, so far as I can discover, Graves's disease does not occur in animals, which fact leaves open the possibility that the exophthalmos produced in them differs in pathogenesis from that of Graves's disease in man.

In human Graves's disease there are two categories of eye signs: (1) wide palpebral fissures, lid retraction, and lid lag, due to levator spasm; and (2) swelling of the orbital tissues, which pushes the eyeballs forward and exudes round the globes, causing swelling of the eyelids (Rundle and Pochin[7]). The characteristic limitation in the movement of the eyeballs is interpreted as a result of weakness of the extrinsic muscles, which are the seat of a myopathy, itself an essential part of the total Graves's syndrome. The morbid anatomy, in its gross features, is fairly well known. There is, as Rundle and Pochin clearly showed, an increase in the total fat in the orbit. There is also, at least in the severer stages, an increase in orbital water content. The muscles display, in the more malignant types, a profound and characteristic myopathy.

They are invaded both by fat and by lymphoid elements. What we need now is some biochemical, especially cytochemical, information about this amazing lesion.

It has seemed to me for some years that quantitative data on intraorbital pressure and records of how it is affected by treatment might be particularly illuminating. I was therefore delighted to receive a monograph on clinical orbitonometry with the description of a successful orbitonometer from Dr. A. C. Copper[8] of Leiden. I have since visited his laboratory. Copper's instrument permits the measurement of the backward displacement of the eyeball when any desired pressure is applied to its anterior surface. Such measurements, I am sure, can be accepted as indices of intraorbital pressure. Copper's orbitonometer is at the same time an excellent exophthalmometer, that is, it can be used to measure the exact position of the eyeball in relation to the line connecting the outer bony angles of the two orbits. One measures simultaneously the intraorbital pressure and the degree of proptosis. The proptosis can be assumed to be the result of balance between the forces which tend to push the eyeball out — that is, increased orbital pressure due to swelling — and the forces which tend to pull it back — that is, the tug exerted by the muscles. Whatever the actual strength of these opposing forces, it must be assumed that, when the position of the eyeball, proptotic or otherwise, is unchanging, these forces must be equal.

Copper reports orbitonometric data on normal people, and in Graves's disease and acromegaly. I quote from his conclusions as follows:

"In thyrotoxicosis and classic Graves's disease orbital tension was either normal or increased. An increase was more evident in eight postoperative cases. The curves most likely suggest a state of mild edema of the orbital tissues.

"In the hyperophthalmopathic type orbital tension was markedly increased, like in diffuse infiltration. One of the cases showed a progress to normal in the course of treatment with thyroid extract.

"Both our clinical observations and the orbitonometry results are in accord with Means's concept of a 'spectrum of types or phases within the clinical entity.' Orbitonometry assists in differentiating the types and in diagnosing a possible progression to hyperophthalmopathy."

Copper here refers to my expressed belief that there is no such thing as a type of malignant exophthalmos etiologically distinct from Graves's disease. I was glad to find that he agreed with me. I believe Pochin does also.

Concentration of Thyrotropic Hormone. For the solution of the eye problem of Graves's disease and the larger one of the entire morbid state, determination of the concentration of thyrotropic hormones in body fluids is obviously indispensable.

Rawson and Starr[2] devised a fairly satisfactory method for urine, making use of the effect of injected material on the height of the thyroid cells in chicks. The very limited data which they have obtained indicate that in thyrotoxic Graves's disease there is an increased excretion of thyrotropic hormone in the inactivated form.

De Robertis[9, 10] observed the rapid accumulation of colloid droplets in the apices of thyroid cells after the injection of thyrotropic hormone, and used this as a test for thyrotropic hormone, finding a relation between the number of droplets and the amount of hormone given. In the blood of four out of eight patients with Graves's disease they found an excess of thyrotropin. Two of these exhibited the ocular signs of the hyperophthalmopathic type. Del Conte, using the same cytologic method, also found normal levels of thyrotropin in hyperthyroidism, but in two patients with malignant exophthalmos and hyperthyroidism he found increased concentrations.

D'Angelo and Gordon[11] have revived and improved the well-known amphibian-metamorphosis test, and believe that with it they can estimate the concentration of both the thyrotropic and the thyroid hormones in the serum. They get their tadpoles into a nonmetamorphosing state by starvation, and then inject them intraperitoneally with the test fluid for example. Two observations are then made: the effect on metamorphosis (growth of the extremities) and the effect on the tadpole's thyroid gland. Thyrotropic hormone causes metamorphosis and hypertrophy of the thyriod epithelium; thyroid hormone also causes metamorphosis but it leads to atrophy of the thyroid epithelium. D'Angelo and Gordon also found normal concentrations of thyrotropin in the blood of patients with ordinary Graves's disease. In two out of eight patients with prominent eye signs there was a modest increase in the blood concentration, but, oddly enough, this increased slightly when desiccated thyroid was administered. Only a few observations have been made, and it is at present difficult to resolve the inconsistencies. Much more spade work and perhaps an easier and simpler method for blood thyrotropin needs to be devised before the complex pattern of pituitary-thyroid relations will emerge.

End-organ Sensitivity. Even though the evidence is scanty, we may still be permitted to speculate on its possible significance. If the thyroid gland and the orbit were targets to the same tropic hormone they would have to respond in parallel to the level of tropic hormone in the blood, unless one or other underwent a change in end-organ sensitivity. One of the two might develop a resistance to tropic hormone not displayed by the other. Thus the thyroid gland could become inactive while the ophthalmopathy was becoming aggravated. But perhaps thyroid gland and orbit are responding to different tropic hormones, the rates of secretion of which may vary independently. To settle these questions we need more information not only on blood titers of hormones but also on sensitivity of end-organs. Rawson and Starr[2] have contributed some information on the sensitivity of thyroid to thyrotropic hormone; as I said before, they find that, in acting on the thyroid cell, thyrotropic hormone becomes inactivated. Further, the cells of thyroids removed from patients with Graves's disease inactivate more thyrotropic hormones than do those of normal persons. No observations of this kind have been made on patients in the hyperophthalmopathic phase, because in such cases we carefully refrain from thyroidectomy. However, what is really vitally needed is information on the sensitivity of end-organs to the thyroid hormone, and what agents determine it. Almost no facts on these important matters have yet been obtained. How actually does thyroid hormone act on cells, and what potentiates or inhibits such action? To these questions we badly need answers.

Thymus Gland. If now we hold that Graves's disease is a widespread and complicated constitutional disorder, we may next inquire what other endocrine glands besides the pituitary and the thyroid are importantly involved in its morbid mechanism. The thymus is, undoubtedly, but is that an endocrine gland? We know nothing very definite about the role of the thymus save that it is often somewhat enlarged in Graves's disease. Selwyn Taylor tells me he has fed five patients with Graves's disease on fresh calves' thymus and noted a fall in basal metabolic rate and improvement in symptoms, but the data are not sufficient to be conclusive. Then there are the ancient claims of such surgeons as von Harberer and Halsted that thymectomy contributes some benefit. In passing we may note that the thymus plays a part in the alarm reaction of Selye; so too does the adrenal cortex, which, moreover, is a perfectly respectable endocrine gland. Therefore its role in Graves's disease may properly next concern us.

Adrenal Cortex. There is rapidly accumulating evidence of a vitally important balance between the thyroid gland and the adrenal cortex. The hormones of each appear to protect against ill effects of overproduction of the other. Thus Koelsche and Kendall [12] found that adrenocortical hormones exert a sparing

action against the negative nitrogen balance induced by thyroxine, and G. W. Thorn (personal communication) has found that
rats made thyrotoxic with thyroid hormone lose less body weight
and show less increase in heart weight if given adrenocortical
extract than do controls given thyroid hormone alone. Conversely,
Zondek[13] states that thyroidectomized animals survive total adrenalectomy longer than do those possessing thyroids, and it is well
known clinically that patients with hypofunction of the adrenal
cortex are far more sensitive to thyroid hormone than are normal
persons.

The opportunities nowadays for studying the interrelations of
the thyroid gland and the adrenal cortex are abundant, because
we have many tests for the functional activity of both these
organs. The thyroid gland can be tested, for example, by its
response to thyrotropic hormone, to iodine, and to antithyroid
drugs, and the effect of thyroid hormone on targets as expressed
by the basal metabolic rate. We can also measure the avidity of
the thyroid gland for iodine by observing its uptake of radioactive
iodine. On the adrenal side, among other things, we can observe
the responses to the adrenocorticotropic hormone, and we can
identify steroids of adrenal origin in the urine.

I have long been curious about the function of the adrenal
cortex in Graves's disease, and when, in 1945, the late Edwin J.
Kepler spent six months in my clinic, I induced him to apply his
water test of cortical function to patients with the thyrotoxicosis
of Graves's disease. He did this in a few cases, but the results
were equivocal. More recently the eosinophil has made its entry
upon the adrenal stage as an index of cortical function. The
eosinophilic population of normal blood is 100–300 per cubic
millimeter. When cortical function increases through the impact
of adrenocorticotropic hormone, there is a sharp fall in the eosinophil count. One can give the hormone directly to man or animal,
or one can stimulate the pituitary to increase its output of the

hormone by giving adrenalin (epinephrine). If after the administration of either adrenalin or adrenocorticotropic hormone there is no fall in the eosinophil count, the conclusion is that the cortex is incapable of being stimulated.

Studies have been under way for some time on cortical function in thyrotoxicosis and myxedema, and of the effect of treatment in each, making use of the several methods of testing which I have mentioned. The results have for the most part been disappointing because the abnormalities disclosed have not been very impressive. Thus in a group of nine thyrotoxic patients the initial eosinophil counts were normal. Three of these failed to show the requisite 50-percent fall after epinephrine, but one of these was 49 percent. The daily excretion of 17 keto-steroids was lower than normal on the average, but these failed to rise appreciably when the euthyroid state was resumed. One patient had a positive Wilder test before therapy and a normal test after. In short, no entirely convincing evidence of altered adrenal function or responsiveness was obtained. This type of observation, however, does not necessarily show how the adrenal cortex is working, because the altered metabolism, changing the rate of disposal of adrenal-cortical secretion, may mask altered production rates or effects of the hormone as measured by our present-day techniques.

Somewhat better evidence of altered cortical function was found in a large group of myxedematous patients studied by Statland and Lerman. There was quite commonly a considerable lowering of the 17 keto-steroid excretion. These values tended to rise as the euthyroid state was restored. Although initial eosinophil counts were higher than normal, the response to epinephrine was quite normal.

One is tempted to generalize that, when either adrenal cortex or thyroid gland increases or decreases its functional activity, the other does likewise in compensation. The Addisonian characteristically has a low basal metabolic rate, and Thorn tells me that he also has a slow uptake of radioactive iodine — another manifestation of lowered thyroid function. When Kendall's Compound E is given to the Addisonian, his uptake of radioactive iodine becomes normal and his basal metabolic rate rises.

Another item of Thorn's I regard as of extreme interest. In his large series of Addisonians he finds a past history of Graves's disease significantly more often than in any random series of patients. I shall have to leave both thymus gland and adrenal cortex at that. Certainly they deserve intensive study in relation to Graves's disease from every possible angle.

Thyrotoxic Crisis. The thyrotoxic crisis, or thyroid storm, also deserves intensive study. This remarkable event in the course of Graves's disease was formerly far commoner than it is today and may be the "Open Sesame" to the conundrum of Graves's disease. The best guess that I can make about its significance is that it may represent what we may call decompensated Graves's disease. There is an acute failure in the ability of the body to adjust to the thyrotoxicosis; a breakdown occurs, with the fulminating development of hyperthermia. I can see some analogy between it and the hyperthermia of sunstroke. The opportunity to study thyrotoxic crisis but rarely presents itself, and when it does is apt to be lost, because so urgent is the patient's situation that all efforts are directed toward treatment, and investigation goes by the board. I urge any of those who encounter such cases to mobilize all aid possible and obtain all the facts possible about the levels of hormones and electrolytes in body fluids. For example, there is hardly any information about the variations in the protein-bound iodine in the serum in the course of thyrotoxicosis. We would expect that this might rise sharply and concomitantly with the crisis, but this is not necessarily so, and many of the features of thyrotoxicosis might be explicable in terms of hypo-adrenocortism, or perhaps in some other way.

Thyroidectomy. As regards primacy, or lack of primacy, of the

thyroid gland in Graves's disease, the usual effectiveness of ablation of that organ, whether by surgery, drug, or radiation, is in-
triguing. Many years ago J. de J. Pemberton, of the Mayo Clinic,
remarked to me that the results of subtotal thyroidectomy were
better than theoretically they should be. If the morbid cause is
left behind, why does not the disease invariably recur after operation? Sometimes it does, but more often it does not. Pemberton
suggested that a hormonic vicious circle has been set up in some
way in Graves's disease and is broken by thyroidectomy, permit-
ting restoration of normal hormonic balance.

Heredity. The role of heredity is a high-priority question. To
assess its importance we need the help of the geneticist, and a
geneticist is already at work on the problem at University College Hospital. Linnell and Greene,[14] at the London County Coun-
cil Thyroid Clinic, have emphasized the importance of the genetic
approach to the etiology of thyrotoxicosis, and Bartels[15] favors
the hypothesis that Graves's disease is a disturbance of balance in
the relations between the thyroid, the vegetative nervous system,
and the pituitary, which, if I understand him aright, is essentially
the theory that I hold. He further believes that in many cases the
disease must develop on the basis of an inherited defect, which
he thinks may reasonably be located in the thyroid. Indeed, in
his opinion Graves's disease is "always due to a genotypic disposi-
tion."

Epidemiology. Another clue may lie, I believe, in the fact that
Graves's disease, at times, is epidemic. In his last paper on the
Danish epidemic Meulengracht[16] indicates that the spot map of
cases bears a striking resemblance to that of an infectious disease.
He does not go so far as to conclude that Graves's disease is infectious, but he does submit that here is a resemblance which
requires explanation. I agree on this last point, but I cannot yet
bring myself to believe that infection is a causal factor in Graves's
disease. It has no other characters that I am aware of that suggest
an infectious origin.

CONCLUSION

I surmise that Graves's disease is somewhat analogous to the adaptation syndrome of Selye[17] except that it is pathological. Perhaps tentatively we might call it a "maladaptation syndrome" and look on it as a type of response that persons of certain constitutional pattern make when they encounter certain adverse circumstances in living.

5 The need for iodine

It may be stated as absolute truth that neither man nor any of his fellow creatures who possess thyroid glands, nor perhaps others, for all I know, are able to live out their normal life span in the total absence of iodine. This element they must receive from their environments, but the amount they need is amazingly small. This small quantity is needed by the body for just one purpose, the completion of the biosynthesis of thyroid hormone. Without iodine no physiologically active thyroid hormone can be built, and without thyroid hormone a normal life cannot be lived. When faced with a shortage of iodine, however, the body can effect certain adaptations which permit great economy in the use of this essential substance.

Let us start with cases. The portrait shown in Fig. 8 was kindly given me by my friend, Dr. Elwood Sharp, Director of Research of Parke, Davis & Company. It was taken by one of their people in a field study in the Peruvian Andes. The subject of the portrait is a denizen of that region, let us call him Francisco. He appears to have something unusual in his neck, but since he has his hat and shirt on, we may conclude that it does not prevent his getting about a bit, nor judging by his facies is his general health or equanimity disturbed in any way.

We need not belabor the question of what this mass is. Obviously it is an enormously enlarged thyroid, or, in common parlance, a goiter. I can think of nothing that could even remotely resemble it except Hodgkin's disease, and this lesion really bears only a very superficial resemblance to Hodgkin's. The anatomic parts of the thyroid, though grossly swollen, are preserved and easily discernible. The right lateral lobe is the larger and is divided in two, giving it a dumbbell shape. The left lobe is more nearly in one mass, and the so-called isthmus connecting the two is plainly visible. In the picture I cannot detect the pyramidal lobe, but that is hardly to be expected. Over the surface of the mass there is easily to be seen a tracery of large veins, which suggests that a great quantity of blood must be emerging from this monstrous organ. One of the criteria by which one judges whether any mass in the neck is thyroid, is that if so, it should rise during the act of swallowing. But if Francisco could raise his by swallowing, I could only say, he is some swallower! Since so far as we know he is still contentedly carrying it about with him, we can but guess as to its weight. My guess would be 2 kilograms or more — the weight of the normal thyroid gland being a mere 20–30 grams. Surely it is as big as some newborn babies, and it looks as much like a baby as some modern sculptures look like human beings.

With that shut mouth of his, Francisco does not appear to be having any difficulty in breathing, nor did the original colored photograph indicate any degree of cyanosis. Yet because the thyroid is attached to the trachea, one might wonder why a lesion of this character does not produce suffocation. The answer is that it hangs downward and outward in front of the chest, actually pulling away from the trachea instead of pressing upon it and occluding it.

We can speculate with some confidence about the anatomy of this goiter, because many like it have been examined. It is undoubtedly made up chiefly of solid nodules and cysts, both varying in size from the microscopic up to golf- or tennis-ball size. The solid nodules will be of any (or all) of the common types of benign thyroid adenomata. Probably there is no malignant tissue in it. The cysts will contain material which in consistency may run from thick jelly or cheesey material to clear liquid, and may

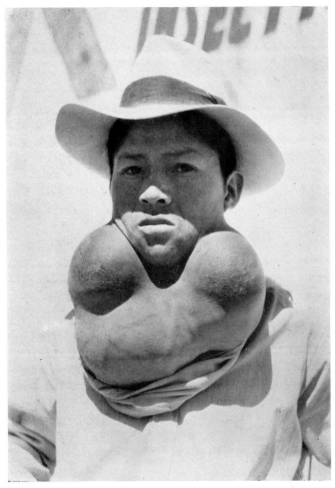
Fig. 8. "Francisco"; endemic goiter from the Peruvian Andes. (Courtesy of Dr. Elwood A. Sharp of Parke, Davis & Company, Detroit, Michigan.)

vary in color from pale watery to dark brown or black — the result of old hemorrhage. Some of the cysts may be very thin walled. There will be much coarse trabeculation with thick fibrous tissue, and scattered throughout there will be islands of parenchymal tissue, micro- or macrofollicular, some with high columnar epithelium resembling the hyperplastic thyroid tissue of Graves's disease. The epithelium of the larger follicles and cysts will be very low.

And so we come to the question of just what a goiter of this type represents. What is its pathogenesis? We cannot answer this question without taking geography into consideration. This subject of ours, Francisco — I cannot call him patient because he has sought no medical advice — merely posed for a picture. Actually he accosted our friend and asked for a match to light his cigarette. The match was supplied in exchange for a snapshot. Very likely the last thing Francisco would want to do would be to part with his goiter. Many people are reluctant to part with such features. They may be their chief or only claim to distinction. The point is, however, that where he comes from many people have goiters. The condition is, in fact, as we say, endemic.

There are various endemic goiter regions in the world, and their approximate location is shown in Fig. 9. A very low concentration of environmental iodine is characteristic of all of them, and it is now very generally believed that therein lies the cause of endemic goiter. It is the thyroid gland's response to iodine want. Other theories of the cause of endemic goiter have been advanced, but it is noteworthy that at an international conference on endemic goiter throughout the world, held at Mill Hill near London under the auspices of the World Health Organization in December 1952, no serious objection to the iodine-want theory was raised. My colleague, Dr. J. B. Stanbury, participated in this conference and has given me a first-hand account of it.

The map shown in Fig. 9 was produced by the Chilean Iodine Educational Bureau. Chile, being the source of much of the

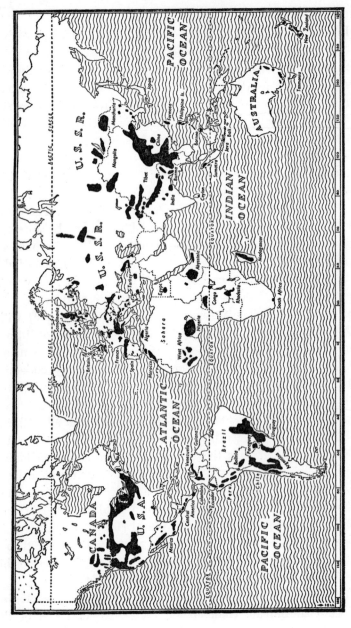

Fig. 9. Endemic-goiter map of the world. (Courtesy of the Chilean Iodine Educational Bureau.)

world's iodine, is eager to find markets for its product, whether
the purpose be goiter prophylaxis, rain-making, or other. The
black areas in this map are for the most part either mountainous
regions or old glaciated areas, these being the types of terrain
from which most of the iodine has been washed out and carried
through the rivers to the sea. The map, of course, although the
best available, is but a first approximation. For one thing it does
not indicate the severity of the endemic in any area, whether
severe, moderate, or mild. For another it does not indicate the
accuracy of data. For certain areas, for example, Switzerland, the
United States, Scandinavia, or New Zealand, there is very exact
information, while for certain remote regions the blackened areas
represent little more than guesswork. Furthermore, the map is
not up to date, because in certain areas the endemics have been
largely eliminated by goiter prophylaxis, as in Switzerland and the
United States, for example.

The prevention of endemic goiter as far as the biological aspect
of the matter goes is very simple. In regions where the natural
iodine supply is below the needed minimum, artificial supply of
an adequate amount of iodine to all persons will in course of
time ensure a goiter-free community. I say in course of time,
because no amount of added iodine would make go away such
a goiter as Francisco's. Although such a lesion is directly due
to iodine lack, the fact remains that when it attains a size and appearance anywhere near approaching this one, it has long since
become an irreversible affair. Therefore the inauguration of a
goiter-prophylaxis program only prevents new goiters from being
formed in children and adolescents. The only way by which the
preëxisting well-established goiters can be got rid of is by the
knife of the surgeon or the death of their possessors. I will speculate as to what determines irreversibility a little later when I
describe the anatomical development of such lesions.

Various methods of administering iodine in a goiter-prophylaxis
program so that everyone will receive his proper quota have been

tried. I think it fair to say that the use of iodized table salt is now generally conceded to be the most effective. The quantity of iodine (1:100,000 minimum) that need be added to table salt is very small. I will return to that matter after I have considered the metabolism of the element.

If endemic goiter is purely a difficiency disease — difficiency of iodine — and I believe that to be the case, then it should be possible to eliminate it throughout the whole world. It was in the belief that this can be done that the World Health Organization called the Mill Hill Conference. There are, however, great difficulties, and they lie in the realm of education as to need, and of distribution in backward or remote communities. It is not a simple problem, for example, to get iodized salt into all the inhabitants of the hill country of Tibet, the jungles of Africa, or the plateaus of central China.

Why should iodine lack produce a goiter of the size and character of Francisco's? To answer this question we must first take notice of how the body uses iodine in health. The metabolic cycle is now fairly well known. In delineating it, both chemical methods and the use of radioactive isotopes of iodine have been necessary. Iodine enters the body chiefly via the alimentary canal in food, drink, or perchance as medicine, although small amounts may be inspired and absorbed by the lungs. In the event that tincture of iodine is painted on the skin, some iodine may be absorbed by that route also. We need, however, concern ourselves with ingested iodine only, which is, under the circumstances of normal living, the only channel of any importance.

Iodine may enter orally as iodide, iodate, or iodinated amino acids, in various stages of linkage. Pure thyroxine might be given orally by a doctor, although there is little sense in that, or an iodinated protein of some sort might enter as food.

Following digestion, iodine is absorbed largely from the intestines and reaches the plasma, regardless of its original state, as iodide. By diffusion iodide reaches all fluids of the body and comes into equilibrium with the plasma.

There are several organs which continually remove iodide from the plasma, one which withdraws it for manufacturing purposes, the thyroid gland, and several, chiefly the kidneys, which withdraw it for excretory purposes. Besides the kidney, the salivary and sweat glands excrete iodide. A small amount of hormonal iodine gets into the liver and is excreted in the bile and lost in the feces, and a very small amount may appear in the urine. The renal excretion is by far the most important of the excretory pathways, and it may be correctly said that after iodide reaches the plasma, the kidney and the thyroid gland come into competition for it. The thyroid must collect what it needs before the kidney has thrown it out with the body's other waste products. In simple terms, then, such is the fate of inorganic iodine in the body, either to be excreted by the kidney or collected by the thyroid. What leaves the kidney has left the body permanently, and what is collected by the thyroid is synthesized into organic forms of iodine, and leaves the thyroid only in amino acid combination.

The utilization of iodine by the thyroid cells to make thyroid hormone has been discussed in the second of this collection of lectures. Suffice it to say here that the gland appears specifically to trap such quantity of iodide from the blood which passes through it, to make such quantity of hormone, as the body requires for its total metabolic economy. The steps in the process briefly are, first, oxidation of iodide to iodine, next, iodination of tyrosine to diiodotyrosine, and finally, coupling of two diiodotyrosines to form a single molecule of thyroxine. Thus begins what may be called the organic cycle of iodine in the body. Entering the thyroid gland as iodide, iodine leaves the thyroid largely as thyroxine. However, there is an inner cycle in the organic iodine pathway. Unique among endocrine glands, the thyroid is not only a factory making its hormone, but also a warehouse which can store the hormone.

Let us now trace the rest of the organic cycle. Thyroxine when fabricated by the thyroid cells is delivered to the follicular lumena of the gland and stored there as thyroglobulin. As thyroxine is needed, thyroglobulin is broken down and delivered to the blood stream, in which it probably travels bound to plasma proteins, finally to reach its target cells, namely, all tissue cells of the body.

What happens when thyroxine reaches its target cell is not yet known. It gains entry to the cell somehow, and presumably enters into, or conditions in some way, the oxidative reactions or energy-storing reactions of the cell. It now appears likely that in order to accomplish this result it must first be converted to triiodothyronine, and that it accomplishes its hormonal action in that form. Further researches by cytochemists will be necessary to solve these mysteries. It may be said in passing that recently a patient at the Massachusetts General Hospital with complete myxedema was given 100 micrograms of triiodothyronine daily for 14 days, and made a calorigenic response quite like those commonly obtained with 500 micrograms daily of thyroxine.

The hormone having served its purpose, its remnants become metabolites, calling for excretion. The iodine they contain is reduced to inorganic iodide, and is added to the general iodide pool available to the thyroid. Thus the thyroid has two possible sources of iodide, that derived from the metabolism of thyroxine and that newly received from external sources.

The body has learned to deal with iodine very economically. The amount of thyroxine iodine which must be produced by the thyroid to keep the average human in a euthyroid state is in the neighborhood of 50 to 100 micrograms of hormonal iodine per day (thyroxine is 60 percent iodine). Because of the body's ability to reuse iodine, however, perfect health can be maintained on iodine intakes lower than that.

In most nongoiterous regions the daily ingestion of iodine is far in excess of the minimum requirement. The average excretion of iodine, which may be assumed to approximate the intake, may be, without added iodide, in such places as the eastern seaboard of the United States, between 100 and 200 milligrams per day, and when iodine is given as medicine, as it used to be to a greater extent than now, quite fantastically high excretions may be encountered.

An intake of iodine, however, over and above the thyroid gland's proper needs, has no effect on thyroid function in the normal subject. At any level of iodine supply above the minimum requirement, the gland merely traps what it needs and lets the rest go to the kidney for excretion. No increased output of thyroxine is caused, except in iodine starvation, by raising the intake of iodine. The only effect of a large intake of iodine is that sometimes in certain subjects iodine causes toxic reactions, generically known as iodism. Probably an allergic factor is concerned in the production of these manifestations.

As iodine intake falls, no inconvenience to the thyroid gland results until a point is reached considerably below the rate of output from the gland of thyroxine iodine, 40 micrograms perhaps. Below this point certain compensatory adaptations have to be made in order that the state of euthyroidism may be preserved. And that brings us back to Francisco. In the region he comes from, iodine is a scarce element, and, judging by what has been found in persons resembling him, and similarly situated, we may guess that his urinary output of iodine is not above 5 to 10 micrograms per day. It may be even less than that. He is suffering from a high degree of iodine starvation, but he isn't letting it bother him much.

Why, however, does iodine starvation make Francisco's thyroid swell up to something like the size of a newborn baby? It was to throw some added light on this question that the Thyroid Clinic of the Massachusetts General Hospital sent an expedition to study the goiter endemic in the Andes of Argentina. I had for many

years dreamed of making a goiter tour of the world, but a sufficient detonating stimulus did not arrive until a day in the fall of
1950, when a visitor to the clinic from Argentina, Dr. Hector
Perinetti, Professor of Surgery at Mendoza, pulled out of his
pocket a sheaf of photographs showing a lot of people closely
resembling Francisco. "We should send an expedition to Mendoza
to study these patients by modern methods," said I. "God, when
do we start," said my young colleagues.

The upshot of this rencontre was that in the summer of 1951
Stanbury, Riggs, and Brownell — clinician, pharmacologist, and
physicist — proceeded to Mendoza, armed with Geiger counters,
radioiodine, and various other necessary gadgets, and joined
forces with Perinetti, Del Castillo, and Itoiz to study patients with
endemic goiter.

A preliminary report of their findings has already been published,[1] both in English and in Spanish, and the full and detailed
account is now in press.[2] From the point of view of the
present discussion, one of the most important findings was that
the avidity of the thyroid for iodine bears an inverse ratio to the
supply of iodine available to it. For example, the thyroid of a
normal human in a nonendemic-goiter area will, when a standard
tracer dose of radioactive iodine is administered, pick up about
20–50 percent of it. In such an area if more than 50 percent of
the tracer dose is collected by the thyroid, such a high rate of
collection would be interpreted as strong evidence that the subject is thyrotoxic. However, it was found by the Andean goiter
expedition that in iodine-poor Mendoza persons with goiters resembling Francisco's would collect more than 90 percent of the
tracer dose and still show no evidence whatever of being thyrotoxic. They were euthyroid or occasionally even hypothyroid.
In other words, as the thyroid gland is progressively starved of
iodine, its ability to collect iodine progressively increases. And in
that fact lies part of the explanation of why, in an endemic-goiter
region, the size of the thyroid gland increases.

The total iodine content of the 20–30 milligram thyroid of a normal human subject living in an environment with adequate supply of iodine is in the neighborhood of 5–20 milligrams. This may be regarded as the iodine-storing capacity of such a normal gland. Should a great excess of iodine be administered to such a subject, the iodine content of the thyroid would not rise. The total iodine content of a goiter like Francisco's, on the other hand, despite its colossal size, is smaller than that of the 20-gram gland. It might be no more than 1 milligram. If one presents such a goiterous gland with an abundance of iodine, it will collect it furiously up to a total content of as much as 50 milligrams or more. Stringency of iodine has greatly enhanced its avidity for iodine, and this adaptation is obviously related in some fashion to the greatly increased size of the gland.

The total mass of the thyroid gland, if we exclude stroma and blood and extracellular fluid, is separated into parenchyma and colloid — factory and warehouse. In a gland such as Francisco's there is a great increase in both these components.

In describing the probable anatomical structure of Francisco's goiter I predicted that one would find a considerable increase in thyroid parenchyma, that is to say, hypertrophy of thyroid cells and hyperplasia of the parenchymal tissue. It was shown many years ago by Marine[3] that such is the first anatomical response of the thyroid gland to iodine want, and, after all, when one stops to think, it is quite what might have been expected.

I like to draw an analogy to a smelting plant. The operator of this plant is under contract to deliver refined metal at a certain rate. He has a supply of high-grade ore, sufficiently large so that his plant working to full capacity can produce the required metal. Now let us suppose he is suddenly no longer able to obtain high-grade ore. Under the new circumstances only low-grade ore is available to him. What does he do? Either he fails to meet his contract or he takes steps to accomplish his objective despite the decline in the quality of ore. One way to do this would be to increase the size of his plant. That seems to be what the thyroid does when faced with a decline in its iodine resources. When an adequate iodine supply is restored to such a hyperplastic gland, the thyroid cells themselves may be expected to recede to a normal status, and consistent with such expectation is the clinical fact that under iodine therapy early stages of endemic goiter are indeed reversible.

Goiters such as Francisco's, however, are not at all reversible, and that is because included in their huge size is not only an increased volume of parenchyma, but also a huge increase in the amount of colloid material and the products of its degeneration stored in the follicles. There is a warehouse problem as well as a factory problem in goiters of this type.

The explanation of the colloid storage excess is not as evident, to me, at least, as that of parenchymal hyperplasia. Under the drive to extend the parenchyma when faced with iodine want, which no doubt is exerted through increased thyrotropic action of the pituitary, the thyroid cells presumably increase their output of thyroid protein even when they cannot properly iodinate it. That results in a progressive stuffing of the follicular lumina with colloid, and their getting bigger and ever bigger so long as the individual remains in a state of iodine want. Such colloid, because of its poverty of iodine, is useless as a source of hormone. Apparently it stays permanently in the follicles, and, so to speak, rots there. So far as I am aware, no agent has yet been found that will mobilize it once it has piled up in this fashion. Proteolytic enzymes have been found in the thyroid, but they do not seem to be available to cause dissolution of such colloid as Francisco has stored, even should he be given an abundance of iodine. What would probably happen to Francisco if he were given iodine would be that his extensive and iodine-hungry thyroid parenchyma would seize upon it and convert it to thyroxine at a rate far in excess of his body's requirement of hormone, and thus he would go into a state of hyperthyroidism. This sort of sequence

of events, never seen in nonendemic-goiter regions, is what years
ago the Swiss called Iod-Basedow.

In order to obtain a somewhat more vivid impression of these
various relations and adaptations of iodine metabolism I would
like now to make use of some diagrams which Riggs[4] has prepared on the basis of observations made at Mendoza, and from
other sources. For his own purposes of mathematical analysis,
Riggs simplified the iodine situation (I have still further simplified it for my own purposes) by assuming that all the iodine in
the body falls into one of three compartments, namely, inorganic
iodide (the iodide pool), organic iodine in the thyroid gland,
and organic iodine in the blood and extrathyroidal tissues. He
represents them diagrammatically by cubes, the volume of each
cube being proportional to the quantity of iodine within the
compartment which it represents. The pathways from one compartment to another are indicated by arrows, and the width of
each arrow is proportional to the quantity of iodine traversing it
per unit time. In this way the impression is given a quantitative
flavor. It must be remembered, however, that it is also a simplified
one — we will hope not oversimplified.

Figure 10 indicates the state of affairs in a euthyroid person
living in an iodine-sufficient area. As thus represented, the quantity of organic iodine in the thyroid is about 90 times that in the
iodide pool, and 16 times that of organic iodine elsewhere. The
diagram also indicates that there are two main currents of iodine
flow in such a system. There is the in-and-out one of mouth–pool–
urine, and the circular one of pool–thyroid–tissues–pool. Under
the circumstances of Fig. 10, the mass movement of iodine along
the former is about double that around the latter. If a dose of
iodine were fed the subject, the in-and-out flow would be increased, but not the circular.

In Fig. 11 are represented the relations in an iodine-starved
person. The in-and-out current has shrunk to a mere trickle. So

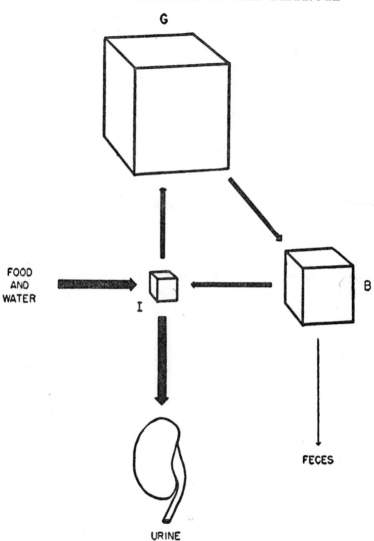

Fig. 10. Metabolism of iodine in a euthyroid subject living in a region with adequate iodine supply. The cube I represents the quantity of iodine in the iodide pool; cube G, organic iodine in the thyroid gland; and cube B, organic iodine in the blood and body fluids. The width of the arrows indicates the volume flow of iodine between compartments. (After Riggs.)

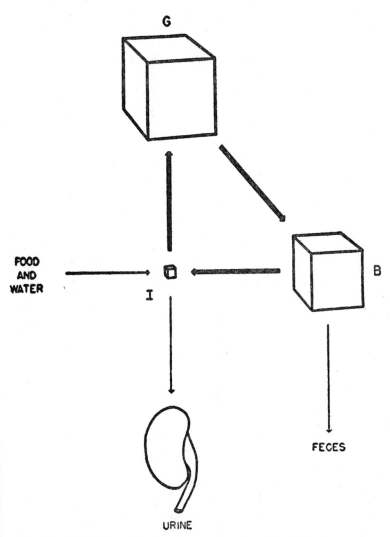

Fig. 11. Metabolism of iodine in a euthyroid subject living in a region where iodine supply is inadequate. (After Riggs.)

has the iodide pool, but through reutilization of iodide of metabolism, and the development by the gland of the ability to collect
iodide from very low concentrations, sufficient output of hormone
is maintained to keep blood and tissue organic iodine (that is
to say, hormone iodine) at a normal level, and thus keep the
subject in a euthyroid state. If the time ever came when the thyroid gland sucked the iodide pool dry, so to speak, then at last
the subject would pass into a hypothyroid state.

If the body were iodine-tight in the way it is iron-tight, then,
having once been charged with a sufficient store of iodine, it
could carry on with no renewal, merely using the same iodine
over and over. But the body is not so constructed. It loses some
iodine, and therefore, though it can economize, it cannot do
without.

There are a couple of other considerations brought up by a
goiter like Francisco's: first, the question of whether any factor
other than iodine want play a role in the production of such a
goiter as his, and second, whether there is any such thing as
acclimatization to iodine want.

When I was young there was a theory that endemic goiter was
due to drinking water from melting snow. There was some truth
in this, but it was merely that water from melting snow contains
little or no iodine (at least from the snow of the high mountains).
There have also been theories that calcium played some part, but
it is my belief that the only factors other than absolute iodine
want that enter into the genesis of endemic goiter are substances
of the cyanide or thiourea groups which act in an indirect way.
The point about such substances is that they place an impediment
to the thyroid's collecting, or utilizing, iodine to make hormone.
If such agents occur widely in an endemic-goiter region, they
will tend to intensify the process, though I doubt if they often are
the primary cause. In the presence of such goitrogenic agents it
takes a larger dose of prophylactic iodine to prevent the develop-

ment of goiter than were they not present. They act as adjuvants to the morbid process, not as primary cause.

As to acclimatization, there is but scant evidence. There are some accounts of a higher degree of goiterousness in new arrivals to an endemic-goiter region than there is among the natives. It is not difficult to believe that a greater power to consume iodine might be developed by the thyroids of persons long exposed to iodine want than among new arrivals. Such adaptations would be analogous to the high red-cell counts one finds in the dwellers at high altitudes, and their greater ability to withstand the effects of anoxemia. To what extent there is such a thing as acquired resistance to aniodemia, I do not believe is known.

And now finally I have to make a few points collateral to our main topic.

The first is the highly puzzling finding that goiters anatomically indistinguishable from Francisco's may occur sporadically in non-goiterous areas, and in the absence of any excess of external goiterogenous substances. What they represent is by no means obvious.

Undoubtedly there is such a thing as intrinsic iodine want, a block to the use of iodine somewhere along the biosynthetic pathway. Examples of this were mentioned in Lecture 2 (see page 26). Under such circumstances the subject ultimately reaches some degree of hypothyroidism — sporadic goiterous cretinism we may call it. Such a situation is explicable. However, when one finds goiters like Francisco's in nongoiterous regions, and with no evidence of an inadequacy of thyroid function, then indeed there is occasion for mystification. What the large goiter in the presence of abundant iodine supply, and with complete euthyroidism in the subject, represents, I do not believe is known. It presents a fine subject for research.

The nature of the peculiar action of iodine in Graves's disease is also a sixty-four dollar question in thyroidology. If one gives

iodine to a person like Francisco, he is likely to become thyrotoxic, but if one gives it to a patient with Graves's disease who
is already thyrotoxic, his thyrotoxicosis is relieved. In both persons
there is hyperplasia of the thyroid parenchyma, and in both the
giving of iodine causes anatomic involutions, but in one case
thyroid-hormone secretion is raised, in the other it is lowered,
through the administration of iodine. In other words, giving an
excess of iodine, which has no effect on the functioning of the
normal thyroid gland, has a very striking effect on the gland in
Graves's disease. The thyroid in Graves's disease is under some
pathologic urge to overfunction. An excess of iodine allays this,
but how or why remains a problem.

In conclusion I will revert to endemic goiter, and raise the
question, do such lesions inflict upon their owners any injury? If
the people in an area like Francisco's do not object to having
goiters, is there any justification for forcing a goiter-prophylaxis
program upon them? Sir Charles Hercus of Dunedin, New Zealand, where they have a considerable endemic area, told me that
some difficulties were encountered when the government first
tried to enforce the sale of iodized salt. The independent New
Zealander felt his rights were being invaded if he were forced
to use iodized salt even for his own good. They got around that
difficulty by providing both iodized and noniodized salt. If a
customer does not expressly ask for the noniodized, he gets iodized salt, and, under those circumstances, very few ask for noniodized. Thus a fairly effective prophylaxis program is under way
in that country and everyone is happy about it.

The point is, however, that there are more weighty reasons
than the cosmetic for the eradication of endemic goiter. As an
endemic persists and runs through successive generations, there
is a cumulative factor of thyroid insufficiency which produces
increasing numbers of persons in whom the economy of iodine
usage no longer suffices to maintain the euthyroid state. When

infants are born to hypothyroid mothers, they themselves are hypothyroid from birth or earlier. Thus in all the severe endemic regions of the world, not only are there euthyroid persons with large goiters such as Francisco, but also many stunted and imbecilic goiterous dwarfs resulting from intrauterine iodine lack, the so-called cretins, well known for centuries in such places as Switzerland. Not only are there classic cretins in these endemic areas, but many partially hypothyroid people, all of whom suffer somewhat in their health and energy because of inadequate thyroid function.

For these several reasons, then, as a public-health measure, goiter prophylaxis is fully justified. A worldwide deficiency disease can now be fully eradicated. To further this purpose the World Health Organization did well to call the London Conference.

REFERENCES

Lecture 1

1. C. S. Sherrington, *The Integrative Action of the Nervous System* (New York: Scribner, 1906).
2. I. P. Pavlov, *Lectures on Conditioned Reflexes* (New York: International Publishers, 1928).
3. W. B. Cannon, *The Wisdom of the Body* (New York: Norton, 1932).
4. W. McDermott, E. G. Fry, J. R. Brobeck, and C. N. H. Long, *Yale J. Biol. and Med. 23,* 52 (1950).
5. U. U. Uotila, *Endocrinology 26,* 129 (1940).
6. E. De Robertis, *Anat. Rec. 80,* 219 (1941).
7. R. W. Rawson, R. M. Graham, and C. B. Riddell, *Ann. Int. Med. 19,* 405 (1943).
8. B. A. Houssay and A. Biasotti, *Endocrinology 15,* 511 (1931).
9. C. N. H. Long and F. D. W. Lukens, *Proc. Soc. Exper. Biol. and Med. 32,* 743 (1935).
10. H. Selye, *Stress — General Adaptation Syndrome* (Montreal: Acta, Inc., 1950).

Lecture 2

1. C. R. Harington, *Proc. Roy. Soc. (London) B. 132,* 223 (1945).
2. C. R. Harington, *J. Chem. Soc.,* Pt. 1, p. 193 (1944).
3. R. W. Rawson, *Ann. New York Acad. Sci. 50,* 491 (1949).
4. R. W. Rawson and W. L. Money, *Proc. Laurentian Hormone Conf. 4,* 397 (1949).
5. J. H. Means, *Thyroid and Its Diseases* (Philadelphia, Lippincott, ed. 2, 1948).
6. C. R. Harington, *Biochem. J. 20,* 300 (1926).
7. C. R. Harington and G. Barger, *Biochem. J. 21,* 169 (1927).
8. J. Gross and R. Pitt-Rivers, *Lancet 1,* 439 (1952).
9. W. T. Salter, *The Endocrine Function of Iodine* (Cambridge, Harvard University Press, 1940).
10. F. A. E. Crew and B. P. Wiesner, *Brit. M. J. 1,* 777 (1930).
11. B. Nièpce, B., *Traité du Goitre et du crétinisme* (Paris, 1851).
12. W. N. McDermott, E. G. Fry, J. Brobeck, and C. N. H. Long, *Yale J. Biol. and Med. 23,* 52 (1950).
13. J. B. Wyngaarden, J. B. Stanbury, and C. H. Du Toit, *J. Clin. Endocrinol. 11,* 1259 (1951).
14. J. B. Wyngaarden, J. B. Stanbury, and B. Rapp, *Endocrinology 52,* 568 (1953).

15. E. W. Dempsey, *Ann. New York Acad. Sci. 50*, 336 (1949).
16. R. E. Goldsmith, J. B. Stanbury, and G. L. Brownell, *J. Clin. Endocrinol. 11*, 1079 (1951).
17. J. H. Means and J. Lerman, *Ann. Int. Med. 12*, 811 (1938).
18. C. Nieman, *Fortschritte der Chemie Organischer Naturstofte* (Vienna, Springer, 1950).
19. J. H. Gaddum, *J. Physiol. 68*, 383 (1930).
20. C. G. Rand, D. S. Riggs, and N. C. Talbot, *Endocrinology 51*, 562 (1952).
21. E. W. Dempsey and E. B. Astwood, *Endocrinology 32*, 509 (1943).

Lecture 3

1. E. C. Dodds and J. D. Robertson, *Lancet 2*, 1197 (1933).
2. W. F. Rienhoff, Jr., *Bull. Johns Hopkins Hosp. 68*, 538 (1941).
3. R. F. Farquharson and A. H. Squires, *Tr. A. Am. Physicians 56*, 87 (1941).
4. M. Heinemann, C. E. Johnson, and E. B. Man, *J. Clin. Investigation 27*, 91 (1948).
5. R. Goldsmith, S. H. Sturgis, J. B. Stanbury, and J. Lerman, *J. Clin. Endocrinol. and Metab. 12*, 846 (1952).
6. A. Querido and J. B. Stanbury, *J. Clin. Endocrinol. 10*, 1192 (1950).
7. W. H. Perloff, L. M. Levy, and A. Despopoulas, *J. Clin. Endocrinol. 11*, 1495 (1951).
8. A. M. Chesney, T. A. Clawson, and B. Webster, *Bull. Johns Hopkins Hosp. 43*, 261 (1928).
9. D. Marine, E. J. Baumann, A. W. Spence, and A. Cipra, *Proc. Soc. Exper. Biol. and Med. 29*, 772 (1932).
10. R. Hunt, *J. Biol. Chem. 1*, 33 (1905).
11. J. H. Means and J. Lerman, *Ann. Int. Med. 12*, 811 (1938).
12. J. B. Stanbury and A. F. Godley, personal communication.

Lecture 4

1. H. S. Plummer, *The Function of the Thyroid Gland* (St. Louis: C. V. Mosby, 1926).
2. R. W. Rawson and P. Starr, *Arch. Int. Med. 61*, 726 (1938).
3. B. M. Dobyns and B. Lennon, *J. Clin. Endocrinol. 8*, 732 (1948).
4. W. T. Salter, *The Endocrine Function of Iodine* (Cambridge: Harvard University Press, 1940).
5. B. M. Dobyns, B. Skanse, and F. Maloof, *J. Clin. Endocrinol. 9*, 1171 (1949).
6. A. S. Warthin, *Trans. A. Am. Phys. 43*, 164 (1928).
7. F. F. Rundle and E. E. Pochin, *Clin. Sci. 5*, 51 (1944).

8. A. C. Copper, *An Introduction to Clinical Orbitonometry* (Leiden: Stenfert Kroese, 1948).
9. E. De Robertis, *Anat. Rec. 84*, 125 (1942).
10. E. De Robertis, *Ann. New York Acad. Sci. 50*, 317 (1949).
11. S. A. D'Angelo, and A. S. Gordon, *Trans. Am. Goiter Assn.* (1949), p. 140.
12. G. A. Koelsche and E. C. Kendall, *Amer. J. Physiol. 113*, 335 (1935).
13. H. Zondek, *The Diseases of the Endocrine Glands* (Baltimore: Wm. Wood & Co., ed. 3, 1935).
14. J. W. Linnell and R. Greene, *Post-Grad. M. J. 23*, 377 (1947).
15. T. D. Bartels, *Heredity in Graves' Disease* (Copenhagen: Munksgaard, 1941).
16. E. Meulengracht, *Arch. Int. Med. 83*, 119 (1948).
17. H. Selye, *J. Clin. Endocrinol. 6*, 117 (1946).

Lecture 5

1. J. B. Stanbury, G. L. Brownell, D. S. Riggs, H. Perinetti, E. Del Castillo, and J. Itoiz, *J. Clin. Endocrinol. and Metab. 12*, 191 (1952).
2. J. B. Stanbury, G. L. Brownell, D. S. Riggs, H. Perinetti, E. Del Castillo, and J. Itoiz, *Adaptation to Iodine Defficiency: A study of endemic goiter* (Cambridge: Harvard University Press, in press).
3. D. Marine and C. H. Lenhart, *Arch. Int. Med. 7*, 506 (1911).
4. D. S. Riggs, *Pharmacol. Rev. 4*, 285 (1952).

INDEX